D0440311

Praise for Kris Holloway's
MONIQUE AND THE MANGO RAINS

"... a tenuous hold on life and health is made achingly real ..."   — *Boston Globe*

"*Monique and the Mango Rains* bypasses our calloused views and leads us to love and laugh with the amazing individuals who live and work in such dire circumstances."
     — *The Atlanta Journal-Constitution*

"Despite Holloway's anger over wrongs seemingly imbedded in the culture . . . she avoids the trap of cultural superiority. Instead, she simply seeks to help those she has come to love . . ."
     — *Minneapolis Star Tribune*

"A poignant and powerful book."   — *Kirkus,* Starred Review

"Holloway's moving account . . . will interest all those concerned about the realities of women's lives outside the industrialized world."   — *Publishers Weekly*

"... the rhythm of life and death in Mali ... shines through all the pages."   — *Library Journal*

"There have been many accounts, mostly by sociologists and anthropologists, of studying people from other cultures. But there have been few accounts of actually being friends with them. Anyone who is curious about what such a friendship feels like from the inside should read this respectful but intimate account of the bond between Kris Holloway and Monique Dembele."
     — Anne Fadiman, Author, *The Spirit Catches You and You Fall Down,*
     winner of the National Book Critics Circle Award

"This funny, poignant book connects us immediately with women in a far-off land; their triumphs become ours, their struggles become ours. It is a tale of the potential of crosscultural friendship and the power of intercultural exchange."
     — Carol Bellamy, Former Director, UNICEF and U.S. Peace Corps

"*Monique and the Mango Rains* is beautifully and frankly written, both an ethnography of Malian health care and a coming-of-age memoir of Peace Corps participation. I entered this book curious about childbirth in rural West Africa, and learned a great deal about gender relations as they shape the meaning of children, development resources, and the many routes to Malian modernity. Like the short, sweet 'mango rains' that punctuate Kris Holloway's story, this text brings inspiration to its readers."
     — Rayna Rapp, Professor of Anthropology, New York University

"Delicious like mangoes in season, you will not be able to put this incredible book down. We witness the stark reality of lives in a third-world country: the fate of babies and young children, of women dying in childbirth. But we are also there for breathtaking descriptions of beauty, generosity, and intimacy."
— Brigitte Jordan, Author, *Birth in Four Cultures, Fourth Edition,*
winner of the Margaret Mead Award

"*Monique and the Mango Rains* is an astounding book. In her brief narrative, Holloway tells an exquisite story of crosscultural friendship, of women's commitment through their work to bettering the lives of other women, and of the contribution that can be made to a third-world society by citizens of the industrialized world when hubris is not part of the equation."
— Marnie Mueller, Author, *Green Fires,*
The Climate of the Country, and *My Mother's Island*

"Kris Holloway's *Monique and the Mango Rains* . . . is one of the few personal accounts that describes the pleasures and frustrations of Peace Corps life, while simultaneously informing the reader of the realities of rural African life with its own particular joys and tragedies."
— Elliot Fratkin, Professor of Anthropology, Smith College

"The story of Monique is the saga of a woman caught in the web of tradition. I hope the book will reach the homes of many in the West so they may know about the lives of their fellow humans battling poverty, underdevelopment, and diseases in parts of Africa. I also hope the book will find its way back to Mali where Monique's contemporaries and fellow Malians would begin to take heart that loving souls exist abroad and their condition is being communicated faithfully and passionately."
— Sulayman S. Nyang, Professor of African Studies, Howard University

"I enthusiastically recommend this book, for it allows the reader to learn about midwifery and women's issues through the lenses of two very different cultures. It is full of warmth and insight, and having it end was like losing a friend."
— Rahima Baldwin Dancy, midwife, author, and childbirth activist

"The acceptance of what comes with being a woman and at the same time how to push for reform . . . in an environment where women, even as victims, are less than equal is captured in the singular sagesse of Monique in Kris Holloway's remarkable memoir."
— Grace Reading Series, Book Club Pick

"This is a truly inspiring story of a friendship between women from different cultures . . ."
— *Midwifery Today*

"Readers will find this memoir emotionally moving, beautifully written, and highly informative."
— *Journal of Community Health*

"The multiple themes and issues voiced in this narrative provide a useful point of dialogue and reflection for many audiences. Although the subtitle and a great deal of the story focus on midwifery, and infant and maternal morbidity and mortality, the narrative goes further. For students or teachers of African studies or anthropology, Holloway incorporates information about kinship systems, religion and witchcraft, familial and traditional power relationships, and decision-making processes that affect marriages, jobs, women's status, childbearing, and community self-help projects." — *African Studies Review*

MONIQUE AND THE MANGO RAINS

MONIQUE AND THE MANGO RAINS

TWO YEARS WITH A MIDWIFE IN MALI

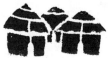

Kris Holloway

John Bidwell
Consulting Editor

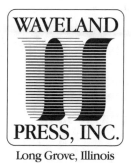

Long Grove, Illinois

For information about this book, contact:
Waveland Press, Inc.
4180 IL Route 83, Suite 101
Long Grove, IL 60047-9580
(847) 634-0081
info@waveland.com
www.waveland.com

literary**ventures**fund

investing in literature
one book at a time

providing a foundation
for writers around the globe

www.literaryventuresfund.org

For Aidan, Liam, Geneviève, Basil, and Christini

Kle di shi kan ma mu

May God give you long life

CONTENTS

ACKNOWLEDGMENTS

There are many people who had a hand in the making of this book, and I want to thank them.

Bill and Jane Holloway, my parents, who encouraged me to go into the Peace Corps, championed my work while I was there, and believed in the ideas of this book long before I put them to paper. My father's photographs appear in the book, and my mother's keen eye for narrative flow, though less noticeable, is distinctly present.

My sister Pam Sheldon, who was there when I most needed her to be, and continues to show unflappable patience for my incessant need to talk even more than I write.

My late uncle Bob Holloway, who was slated to go to Sierra Leone as a volunteer, but went to Vietnam instead. He made the journey to West Africa feel like it was a Holloway destiny.

Those Peace Corps folk, volunteers and staff, who made our experience what it was—challenging and fulfilling—especially Sire Diallo, for logistical as well as moral support; Dawn Camara and Veronica Coulibaly, for their smiles and MIF kits; Julia Earl and Bill Moseley, for connections during our service and during our return trip; Tanya Sisler and Chip Smith, for friendship.

Kay Bork, retired French teacher, who made the French language come alive for me in my early years, and Christian, Christiane, and Lydia Sevette who gave me fluency. Dr. Sam Harrison, retired professor at Allegheny College who taught me to always question assumptions and, therefore, how to think. Carol and Ken Apacki, Patrick and Anne Aubourg, Cass Gowans—dear family friends who opened their homes and hearts to Monique. Eric Romanoff, Bruce Furness, Merle Rockwell, Ira Bates, and Betty and John Bidwell for welcoming Monique during her visit. E. Julian Caldwell, DDS for giving Monique a mouth free of pain.

Irene Butter, Professor Emeritus at the University of Michigan, for her friendship and inspiration, without which I would never have delved so deeply into women's and children's health. Dominique Simon, for access to her anthropological research while she was at the University of Massachusetts and her clarification of many aspects of women's social support systems in Mali.

Midwives Rahima Baldwin Dancy, Merilynne Rush, and Mickey Sperlich, for attending me during the births of my children. And Rahima, for important and insightful comments on the manuscript. Dr. Sangeeta Pati, for her comments on obstetrical care and recovery.

Julie Conley, the volunteer who followed me in Nampossela. Paul Bidwell, Betsy Bartholomew, Sue Brau, Amy Cullen, and Michelle Segar, who never tired (or at least didn't let on that they did) of listening to Monique's story.

Chris Rohmann, writer and reviewer exemplaire who was there in the beginning, and the members of the National Writers Union, Local 5. Dori Ostermiller, Elli Meeropol, Lydia Nettler, Marianne Banks, Brenda Marsian, Rita Marks, Jacqueline Sheehan, Toni Brandmill, and Celia Jeffries—members, current and past, of various incarnations of my writing group that helped finesse this manuscript. They lived through 34 versions of the first chapter and never complained; their grammatical precision and narrative wisdom have made this book an immeasurably smoother ride.

Jane Chelius for her belief in the importance of Monique's story. And for writers Michael Sanders and Aim Russell, for connecting us with Jane. Emily Weir at Mount Holyoke College and Jeni Ogilvie at Waveland Press for their copyediting expertise. Mary Bisbee-Beek, publicity maven, for going above and beyond. My editor Tom Curtin at Waveland for his humor and creative receptivity for a book that didn't fit the mold.

Gretchen Bloom, who has devoted her life to women's health and whose vetting has much improved the ideas represented in the book. Katherine Dettwyler, Elliot Fratkin, Sangeetha Madhavan, Carolyn Sargent, Abdoul Diallo, and Jocie Caldwell-Ryan—reviewers in the academic world who lent their expertise and knowledge, corrected my Bambara, confirmed or corrected my assumptions, and greatly improved the accuracy of the book.

I am especially indebted to my family here in Massachusetts and my family in Mali:

First to my partner in writing and in life, John Bidwell, who never, ever lost faith in this story and my ability to tell it. For his bad puns, buoyant support, and dogged persistence over the years of writing, editing, learning, and research. This book is as much his as mine. To my sons Aidan and Liam, who tolerated me being distracted, sometimes distraught, and always on the computer.

Jean and Apollinaire, Maxim, Didier, Abel, Joseph, and Angel Dembele for welcoming us into the Dembele family, for overlooking and forgiving our frailties and faux pas, and for always keeping that extra bowl or bed for us. Rokiatou Coulibaly, Alima Koné, Sabine Sanogo, and Djeneba Dembele, who helped shed light on Monique's contribution to Nampossela. Kadjatou Keita, the late Mai Keita, and Amadou Gakun for their help being interviewees and interviewers on our return trip. Antoine and Catherine Dembele for their comfort, and especially for the use of Antoine's art throughout this book.

The people of Nampossela who welcomed us in the first time, welcomed our return, and still would welcome us again, especially Bakary and Mawa Dembele, Gawssou Koulibaly, and the late Louis and Blanche Dembele, I am indebted to you all. To Geneviève, Basil, and Christini— thank you for keeping hope alive.

And to all those who I may have forgotten unintentionally . . . thank you.

Note to Reader
Some names have been changed in this story to protect privacy.

REPUBLIC OF MALI

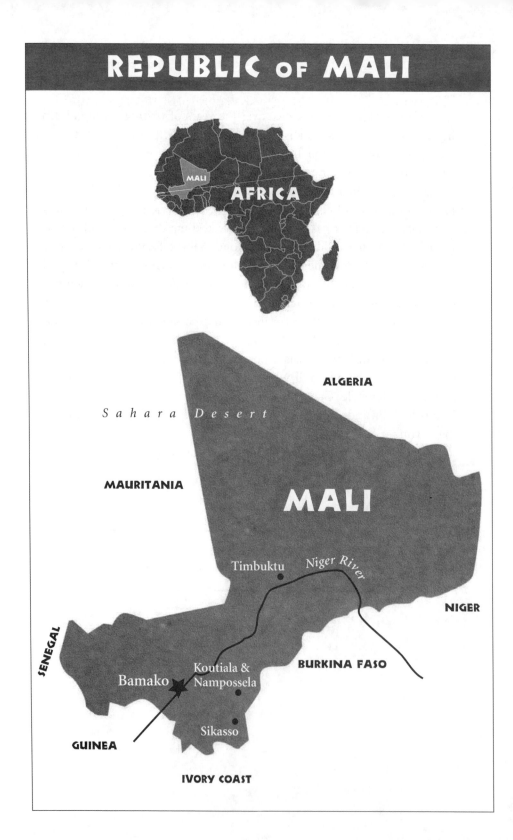

AFRICA

MALI

ALGERIA

Sahara Desert

MAURITANIA

MALI

Timbuktu

Niger River

NIGER

SENEGAL

Koutiala & Nampossela

BURKINA FASO

Bamako

Sikasso

GUINEA

IVORY COAST

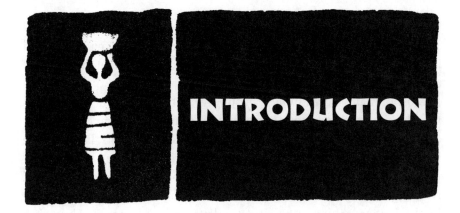

INTRODUCTION

YOUR TWO-YEAR ASSIGNMENT IS IN THE COUNTRY OF MALI, WEST AFRICA. DEPARTURE DATE: JULY 29, 1989. That was the gist of the letter I held in my hands from the Peace Corps, during the spring of my senior year in college. I was twenty-one, ready to escape the Midwest for a few years. Ready for an adventure. And yes, ready to make a difference.

Unlike other Peace Corps recruits, I knew something about Mali. I didn't confuse it with a Hawaiian island. I didn't suffer the disappointment of learning that my two years, although under the sun and near sand, would not be on a beach. My interest and fluency in French, greatly augmented by a semester spent in Paris, had led me to take a little-known course on West African history and civilizations. I learned about Mali's history of trade, gold, and emperors—and of its more recent foray into independence. It was a long way from Ohio, but my parents, my friends, and my favorite professor all encouraged me to go.

Mali is nestled in the center of the great rounded hump that is West Africa. Its present shape and size, which make it twice the area of Texas, are the result of colonial bureaucrats and cartographers. The southern border is wavy, following rivers and hills; the north is long, straight lines that only a vast desert like the Sahara can afford. For centuries, no ossified borders existed at all. Amoeba-like kingdoms expanded and contracted, shifted and sometimes overlapped. Mali is home to Timbuktu, the medieval center of Islamic learning. It is home to Djenne, whose city walls hold the largest and oldest mud brick mosque in the world. It was home to the thirteenth-century kingdom of Mali, ruled by the benevolent king Sundiata

Keita, upon whose story the "Lion King" is based. And it is now a model of democracy for African nations and Muslim countries, having survived French colonialization until 1960 and rule by a military dictator from 1968 until 1991.

Most of Mali's eleven million people live in the south, where the three-month rainy season brings a short respite from the hot temperatures and desiccated landscape. Most of them are farmers and herders, living off the land, sheltering in small mud hut villages, taking their water from wells, their light from oil lanterns, and their food from a pot over an open fire. Ninety percent are Muslim, 1 percent are Christian, and the rest practice local religions, though aspects of the latter infuse them all. Thus, life's rhythms are set by the two most powerful influences in Mali: nature and religion. Muslim prayers mark the hours, and the festivals and rituals of local religions punctuate the year. Rains signal the planting and harvesting, and their absence the time to rebuild and repair.

Mali is one of the economically poorest countries in the world. In fiscal speak this means the average Malian earns $210 US a year. In practical terms this means very few people have electricity, running water, telephones, or cars. They don't have favorite clothes and favorite foods. They wear what they have and eat what is available. They turn to neighbors, Allah, and local gods for help, as there are few hospitals, police, or social services.

There are exports, like gold and cotton, but their economic effects are limited due to generous corruption and lack of infrastructure. And these exports have dark sides. The sudden wealth that accompanies mining towns often breaks ancient traditions and the social fabric of the area. Cotton depletes the soil of nutrients and if not managed properly can destroy croplands. United States and European Union cotton subsidies mean that Malian farmers never get a fair price for their crop.

What Mali lacks in dollars, it makes up for in language and culture. Dozens of languages are spoken. Though Arabic is used for worship, and French is the official language, *Bamanakan* or Bambara, is the true lingua franca and is spoken by almost everyone. Versions of this ancient trade language can be heard throughout West Africa; it is a uniting tongue among the many diverse ethnic groups—the Bambara, Malinke, Sarakole, Peul, Tuareg, Moor, Songhai, Senufo, and one of its subgroups, the Minianka. Bambara is also the native tongue of the Bambara tribe who are part of an ethnic group that comprises half of Mali's population and lives in and around the capital of Bamako. The small and less familiar Minianka tribe populates Mali's southeastern region, near the Burkina Faso border. Arriving in Bamako and heading straight to this region is equivalent to a transatlantic tourist landing in New York City and heading for rural Ohio. It is here among the Minianka that I would live.

From a Westerner's viewpoint, the lives of women in Mali, across all ethnic groups and especially in rural areas, are not easy. Most women are married by the age of eighteen and have seven children (6.8 children, to be exact), one of the highest fertility rates in sub-Saharan Africa. The maternity mortality ratio, or the risk of death during childbirth and pregnancy, is among the top ten highest in the world. Less than 6 percent of women use any type of modern contraception. Over 96 percent have had some form of female genital cutting performed during their infancy or childhood.

These statistics held true for the women in my village, but I didn't know that on the day I joined the Peace Corps. I didn't know that I would meet and befriend Monique Dembele, a village midwife, and spend my two years at her side. I didn't know that I would fall in love with another Peace Corps volunteer. I also didn't know the immensity of the sky when there is nothing to tarnish its glory—unpolluted by electric lights, uncrowded by tall buildings, without a drop of humidity in the air. Nor did I know that my friendship with Monique would continue long after my service was over and that I would return to Mali, after eight years away, to mourn her death in childbirth. Or that I would write a book about our friendship, about her life, and about women's ancient struggles and abiding strengths. I couldn't have known any of this, for all I had was a slip of paper, an invitation to join, a sliver of promise.

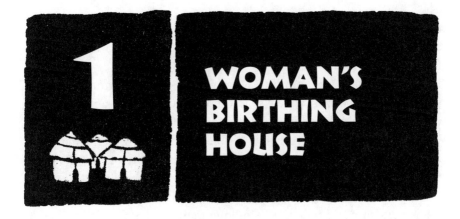

1 WOMAN'S BIRTHING HOUSE

"HOW LONG HAS THE WOMAN BEEN IN LABOR?" I ASKED.

"Since early this morning." Monique's flashlight traced a yellow stain on the dark earth. A scorpion moved under a rock. "I have been with her at the birthing house most of the day."

"So, will she give birth soon?"

"Ah, God willing. You will see; there will be no rest for your Monique tonight."

"How old is she?" I said, jogging a couple of steps to stay next to her.

"Seventeen."

It was a struggle to keep my footing on the rough path through the maze of huts that made up the village of Nampossela. I knew the general direction to the birthing house on the outskirts of town. But the layout of the village remained a mystery, and unless I was accompanied, I tended to run into dead ends or wander in endless circles.

I was glad to be with Monique. In fact, since coming to Nampossela a month before, I was almost always with Monique. She was not only the village's midwife and sole health care worker, but she was also my assigned host. At twenty-four, she was only two years my senior, but I was in awe of her knowledge and ability. As she was one of the few people in the village who spoke French, I constantly peppered her with questions.

"You're sure it is all right if I come along? You know, I have never seen a birth."

"Of course, of course," she said, smiling up at me from beneath her blue sequined headscarf. Her voice always seemed poised to break into a belly-rich laugh. "A woman is always welcome at a birth, Fatumata," Monique explained, using my newly acquired Malian name. "And I am glad your first will be here with me."

Monique's face was youthful, sweet really—a brown symmetrical disk with arching eyebrows, widely spaced eyes, and a slightly upturned nose, making her look like a kid. She was stocky and walked with confidence, her green plastic flip-flops barely visible beneath her wide flapping feet. Strapped to her back with a wide cloth tied over her breasts was her three-month-old son, Basil, fast asleep.

We arrived. Monique opened the door and an overpowering stench made me wince and pull back. Monique went straight in, but I needed to linger outside for a moment in the fresh air. The pale and bloated moon was surfacing through the leaves of a mango tree, casting a faint light on the decrepit building. Above the termite-ridden beams of the doorway was the word *Mùsòjiginniso*. I deciphered the Bambara, "woman come down house"—woman's birthing house. The structure's cement veneer was chipped and failing, revealing mud brick. A corner of the corrugated tin roof gaped, ripped open by a violent storm. Monique had told me that women could no longer give birth here in the rainy season. For the three months that rain fell, she helped women give birth in their huts, sometimes walking many kilometers to get there. I wondered if repairing this place would be a project the Peace Corps would fund.

"Fatumata, where are you?"

I took a deep breath and crossed the threshold, the tin door wobbling as I shut it behind me. I felt as if I was drowning in the smell of flesh, body fluids, and leftover food. Shut tight, the building was like an oven, baking all the secretions and juices into a rank casserole. But here, despite the oppressive heat, women found a rare taste of privacy in an otherwise communal world. In fact, the birthing house was one of the few hallowed grounds where men were not allowed to tread.

Jutting from the left wall and dominating the birthing room was an immense concrete block that served as the delivery table. Its gray bulk, illuminated by a single lantern, suggested a sarcophagus. On top of the bare scrubbed surface a naked woman crouched, strained, and pushed, her black skin shining in the dim lantern light. Another woman sat beside her on the slab, supporting her. The wall behind them had a large, worn, greasy spot where countless backs and heads had writhed and reposed.

Monique stood near them, watching. Folded carefully on the floor lay a large square of colorfully decorated cotton cloth—a *pagne*, the traditional garment that Malian women wrap around their waists as a skirt. Set out beside the dented trunk that served as a supply cupboard was a plastic tub for the afterbirth, a medical kit in a tin box, and a frayed birth ledger. So this was childbirth in rural Mali in the late twentieth century.

Monique came over. Raising her chin toward the woman in labor, she said in a whisper, "Fatumata, this is Kadjatou, and her sister, Alima. She has attended many births."

Alima and I greeted one another in Bambara. Kadjatou did not reply.

"Now you will see the real work of a woman," Monique said, as a contraction seized Kadjatou. "If a woman cries with her first child, she will cry with every other child," Monique had said, more than once. To give in to the pain would be a sign of opposing God's will. This was Kadjatou's first child. Her face was contorted and she swallowed with effort, but she was barely audible. A faint moan slipped from between her lips as her body pushed through the contraction. This had been going on for hours. So much work for such little progress.

Monique stepped outside with a teapot of water and soap. There was a minute of splashing and she returned, shaking her hands dry. With no rubber gloves, she had to keep her hands clean. Her fingers housed rocky outcroppings of knuckle that tapered to carefully trimmed nails. She gradually inserted her right hand into Kadjatou's swollen vulva. Kadjatou grimaced as Monique announced that the cervix was fully dilated. "*A be se k'a na*—The baby can come," she said. She pushed a few items aside in the medicine trunk and emerged with a hypodermic syringe and a vial.

An injection. Watching Monique at her clinic over the past weeks I had noticed that the villagers loved shots. To many of them, shots represent the pinnacle of Western medicine, and Western medicine is good. Almost immediately, Kadjatou's contractions began coming with increasing frequency. They possessed her body and her orifices burst forth water, vomit, and diarrhea. I was alarmed. Was this normal, this sending out of liquid scouts in advance of the baby? How could a woman's body survive? It seemed as though she had expelled all she had, until there was only one thing left inside.

The top of the baby's head began to appear. Little by little, with each contraction, more and more bulged forward. A grimace stretched across

Kadjatou's face as her lower half swelled with energy. Oh my, this is simply not going to work, I thought. Really big peg, really small hole. I will never, never have children.

Monique's face was calm, her eyes focused. She began talking Kadjatou through each contraction, with Alima repeating her words in a whispered echo. "*Akanyi . . . I be se, I be se*—Good . . . you can do it, you can do it." Monique's tone and Kadjatou's pushing were in sync, building up and falling down like surf stroking a beach. Her voice seemed the only connection between them and the outside world. Finally, Kadjatou bore down as if pulled by an invisible force. Monique's voice grew stronger and louder, the words stretching out as Kadjatou's body surged forward and birthed the head. A big, slimy globe covered in dark, wavy hair. It hung there. I held my breath. We waited. Another contraction came, and another, each revealing more of the baby's body, until finally the whole child slipped out. I exhaled deeply and stared at the ginger-colored newborn.

Monique quickly took the baby boy and cradled him in her long, muscled arm. She gently massaged his chest with the palm of her hand, leathery fingers sliding over his fragile skin. Finally he opened his mouth, took his first gasp of air, and wailed. Monique cut the blue umbilical cord and began washing him as he sputtered loud protests. Monique's son Basil awoke on her back and began howling, a fine baritone to accompany the new arrival's soprano. Monique wrapped the baby in a towel and placed him beside the medical kit. As Kadjatou pushed out her placenta, Monique caught it in the plastic tub and began inspecting it to make sure that nothing was left inside the new mother. The babies continued their deafening duet. My mouth hung open. I didn't know what to say or think. My dress stuck to my back, wet with perspiration.

Like smoke, I drifted to the corner of the room and down to my knees. I felt overcome with awe and fatigue. I couldn't believe we all got here this way. I couldn't believe that here, in this dilapidated box, Monique, with a sixth-grade education and nine months of medical training, was birthing babies. Lots of babies. She was responsible for the future of this village. No electricity, no running water, no safety net of ambulances and emergency rooms. I knew that Mali had one of the highest rates of maternal death in the world. I'd read a sobering statistic that placed a Malian woman's lifetime risk of dying in pregnancy and childbirth around one in twelve, compared to a U.S. woman's risk of one in over three thousand. Even if one accounts for the fact that Malian women have many more children than American women, and thus are at risk for more years, the difference in the death rate is still huge. Monique was constantly battling the odds. It was so awful, so miraculous. I wanted to get up and help out, but I couldn't do a thing.

Alima climbed down from the cement block and whispered something to Kadjatou, who pushed herself into a sitting position, then heaved herself off the concrete. Hunched over, she picked up her pagne from the floor and shakily covered herself. She walked past me and out of the room. A thin stream of blood trickled down her inner thighs. Alima walked with her, gripping her arm.

"Monique," I said in desperation, finding the strength to rise from the floor. "Where is Kadjatou going? Isn't she going to take her baby?"

"She's not leaving," Monique explained. She bounced Basil on her back to quiet him. "She must go wash herself now. Her bucket of water is already outside." The bathing area was adjacent to the birthing house—in an old *nyegen* (pit latrine), with a floor that was caving into the hole below. I pictured Kadjatou sitting on a small wooden stool, in the corner, rinsing her body back to life with handfuls of cool water.

"But what about the baby?" I asked, looking at the now-peaceful face peering out of the towel by Monique's kit. He was so small, you could almost forget that he was the reason we were all here.

Monique turned to me patiently. "The mother is tired and she must wash herself, Fatumata." Noticing my worry she added, "She will go into the resting room, and we will give the baby to her."

Monique scrubbed and mopped and straightened. I stared at the lantern's flame twitching behind dirty glass as if it were looking for an escape. A hint of kerosene hung in the air. This was Monique's fourth birth this month; the room would be needed again soon. It was hardly sanitary by Western standards; it was made of mud after all, but she kept it as clean as possible. She moved carefully around the baby, stopped momentarily, and looked at him.

"Really, it's very good," she said. "One doesn't know how a birth will turn out, only God does. *Allah k'a balo, k'a nankan di yan.* We just thank God that we have a new baby."

I heard Kadjatou and Alima going into the adjacent resting room. "Fatumata, take the baby and give him to his mother," Monique said, gently lifting the tiny bundle and offering it to me. I did not move. "Hey, Fatu-ma-ta," she smiled, "you can do it. Your hands were made to hold a baby." She helped me cradle him. I grasped him awkwardly. Yet he felt good. Don't drop him, I cautioned myself.

Carefully, I made my way into the resting room. Moonlight had begun to filter through the ripped tin roof. I could see the outline of Kadjatou. She was on her side, resting on a straw mat placed over the iron frame of the bed. Alima was perched on another rusted bed frame.

I placed the baby at Kadjatou's side. She said nothing, but rested a hand on his body. Monique came into the room with her lantern, wrapped a blood pressure cuff around Kadjatou's arm, and began pumping it up.

Kadjatou looked so young. She was *so* young. And if she didn't die, she might have twenty more years of this, of birthing babies. It might be good in God's eyes. It might be good for the village, and good for the baby. But was it good for the mother?

As the air hissed out of the cuff, Kadjatou finally spoke, her dry voice a scratchy whisper.

Monique translated. "Fatumata, they want you to name the baby."

"What? Me?"

"Yes, they are Muslim and will wait for seven days to name him, but because you are here they also want him to have a Christian name."

"I don't understand."

"They want it, that is all. It's okay." She touched my arm. "Don't worry yourself, Fatumata. Just name the baby. You will give it the right name."

How could I come up with the right name? I knew so little about the culture, about what names mean to people. It seemed like such a responsibility. I thought of the most responsible person I knew.

"I would like to give this baby my father's name, a name from my family," I announced. "William."

Monique translated, pronouncing the name "Weelayum," as if she was speaking through okra sauce. She scrunched up her face, smiled, and said "Weelayum" again.

"Weelayum," repeated Kadjatou and Alima, and they both began to laugh. Monique cackled with pleasure and I joined in, happy and relieved. I had not been much help tonight but knew that as long as I was here, I would help Monique in any way I could.

Helping the village was what I had been placed here by the Peace Corps to do. But I was finding that easier said than done. So far I had spent most of my time watching and listening, and looking for opportunities to practice my rudimentary language skills. Slowly, painfully so at times, I absorbed some words, learned some customs, and got used to my new status as the first and only white person ever to live in this village of 1,400 inhabitants.

I had actually been in the country for four months, the first three being spent at the Peace Corps training site near the capital of Bamako. I had been one of forty fresh-faced volunteers, most of us straight out of college. I had thought about the Peace Corps for years. My kin were service oriented, and I was no different. My grandfather was a minister; my mother and uncle were social workers, my father and aunt, school psychologists. My parents volunteered for everything, the church, Brownies, the school. I also wanted to serve overseas because I had grown up around foreigners, no small feat coming from the corn center of Ohio. Ever since I could remember, my family hosted foreign students from both the local college and the high school. I knew students from Malaysia, Egypt, Lebanon, South Africa, and Switzerland.

In Peace Corps training we were dunked in Malian culture. I loved the immersion, soaking up all the details I could. The right hand is considered clean, the left dirty (why? because there is no toilet paper in Malian villages and the left hand is used to wipe). We were taught how to keep ourselves healthy. Drinking dirty water is preferable to no drinking at all. We were trained in our work: how to give health demonstrations, repair wells, build fuel-conserving stoves, plant trees, and protect the shoots from the ever-hungry mouths of goats. Because I was already fluent in French, I concentrated on developing my abilities in Bambara. The Minianka language was not taught in training, as few of us would be sent to this region, and the dialect varied so much between individual villages that one could not learn one version that worked in several towns. Bambara was the language that crossed these boundaries and I found it fun and easy to learn. The pride I took in my language skills was neutralized by my inability to understand my Yamaha 125—the dirt bike that would be my trusted mode of transportation. Though we were taught how to ride and repair them, I found that whatever I took off the bike to clean or replace found its way back on upside down or backwards, with several pieces still left on the ground.

Up to a third of us would not last our two years of service. Homesickness would take its toll, as would family emergencies, injuries (we could all count on at least one motorcycle accident), and sickness. We were told that roughly 70 percent of all volunteers ended up marrying other volunteers. Maybe not anyone here and now, maybe a few years down the road, but it was a sure bet that at least one or two married couples would emerge from our small group. We all looked at one another with suspicion, a few of us forming the Thirty-Percent Club, dedicated to bucking the trend.

The aspect of immersion that I loved the most was being given a Malian name. All volunteers were given Malian names at the beginning of their service. Fatumata was a common Muslim name, derived from Fatima, a daughter of the prophet Muhammad. I was given the last name of Keita, the name passed down from Sundiata Keita, the leader of the great thirteenth-century Malian empire. When I arrived in Nampossela, the village chief, called the *dùgùtigi*, and the village elders insisted that I must take a Minianka name. Thus I took the surname of Dembele and left my Bambara name of Keita behind. "*U be kelen*—They are the same," the dùgùtigi had said. What is Keita to one is Dembele to another. He was a Dembele. All the chiefs before him were Dembeles. Monique was a Dembele. Her in-laws were Dembeles. Now, I was a Dembele. Fatumata Dembele. I loved the sound of it, the short syllables of staccato consonants flowing into liquid vowels.

As a special newcomer, I was housed in a startlingly symmetrical, crisp red brick structure in the shape of an L, standing like an alien outpost on the western edge of the village. One end of the L was a meeting hall, the other was the *doctoroso* (village health clinic) that Monique operated. The corner was formed by two guestrooms joined by a common space. Built a decade earlier by a Chinese development team, it was meant as a showpiece of fired-brick technology, but the technology was too pricey to catch on. The villagers continued to make their bricks along the banks of a nearby stream, with mud, straw, and dung. The latter was used when the clay content of the mud was not high enough to hold the bricks together.

I was staying here, in one of the guestrooms, until the village could build my own hut. And even when my home was built, I would take my meals with Monique and her in-laws, for they had been chosen by the villagers to be my *jàtigi* (host family). She made sure that I had enough to eat, that I learned my way around Nampossela, and that I woke up early each morning, ready to greet the day.

This daybreak was no different, despite our long night at the birth. My guestroom was cavernous and barren, an echoing chamber that amplified every scratch and breath. The grinding of Monique's skeleton key in the sand-filled lock of the clinic jolted me awake, and I was bolt upright by the time she scraped open the iron door next to mine, slammed it against the brick wall, and braced it with a large rock. Even the sounds of her sweeping, shuffling papers, and checking supplies were deafening. It was 6:30 AM and she was ready for business. I was sure that she was aware of my every movement too.

"*I ni sogoma*, Monique—Good morning to you, Monique," I called out in my hoarse dawn voice. I knew it was not customary to greet people before one washed, but she never seemed to mind.

"I ni sogoma, Fatumata. You are awake?"

"Ah, yes. And I am going to bathe."

It would not be long before a small group of villagers would be waiting on the veranda to be seen by Monique for a variety of ailments, ranging from oozing infections to enervating malaria. I liked to be washed and dressed before they arrived. I untwisted my purple sleeping gown from my thin frame, ran my fingers through my wavy mop of dark brown hair, and slid my feet into blue flip-flops. The air was bone dry, and the tiny thermometer dangling from my backpack said 82 degrees Fahrenheit. I ladled a long cool drink from the clay storage jar, and then grabbed my purple plastic bucket, which I had filled half full with well water the evening before.

I leaned left to counterbalance the weight of my bucket on my way toward my bathing area—a vacant, roofless house fifty yards away. Despite erosion from the rains, the walls were high enough for a modicum of privacy. I ducked inside, piled my clothes along one wall, and dropped my bucket in a corner. By squatting low, I could just avoid being seen by any passersby. My white skin virtually glowed in the sunlight, and I felt like a beacon attracting unwelcome eyes. I scrubbed, splashing water that the parched and dusty ground rapidly devoured.

As I rinsed off the bubbles of antibacterial soap, I noticed streaks of red in the disappearing puddle beneath me. My period. Bad timing. The tin trunk that held most of my belongings, including a six-month supply of tampons and pads, had accidentally been sent north to Mopti. It would be another month before a Peace Corps Land Rover would venture out here *en brousse* (in the bush) to deliver my motorcycle and, hopefully, my trunk. I thought about other possible substitutes for pads. Toilet paper? No, there wasn't any in town; a plastic teapot full of water, called a *salidaga*, and one's left hand were used for wiping. Tissues? No Kleenex here; the standard method was to blow out the side of one's nose. I had nothing.

I walked back quickly, my wet flip-flops flicking mud onto the backs of my legs, like a fenderless bike. I rummaged through my large army duffel, for now the sole container of my worldly goods. I couldn't afford to use one of my three shirts, or one of my few dresses. I managed to create a small pile of absorbency—three pairs of white cotton socks and two bandanas. I lined my underwear with a pair of socks wrapped in a bandana, and put on a dress to hide the bulge. What do the women do here? I wondered.

Monique already had her first patient. A woman sat on the examination slab, a stubbier version of the slab in the birthing house, trying to still her whimpering child. The one window in the small room was directly behind her, its dark green metal slats closed against the rising sun, but I could clearly see the deep cut that ran the entire length of the child's right instep. The swollen flesh pulled the wound open and it wept honey-like pus. As Monique dabbed and scrubbed the wound with iodine, the boy began to scream. Flies buzzed about, settling on the gash as soon as Monique raised her ointment-stained red cloth.

One large tin cabinet stood against the back wall, door slightly ajar. It housed bottles of pills and vitamins, tubes of ointments, and vials of liquid for injections. Monique had explained some of the less familiar medicines to me: Spasfon was for gas, Doxycycline for sexually transmitted diseases, and Nystatin for yeast infections. Injectable serums included Amoxicillin, an antibiotic; Kinimax, used for malaria; and Novocaine, a local anesthetic. Monique reached into the cabinet and grabbed some gauze.

"Hold still, little one," Monique said. Basil, snoozing as always on her back, his large head lolling at an impossible angle, created a shiny smear of drool between her shoulder blades. Her muscled arms flexed as she helped hold the kicking child with one hand, and wrapped the foot in the gauze with the other. She then spoke to the woman at length in Minianka. The child finally quieted in his mother's arms. She placed him on her back, though he was much too big to be carried this way, and left.

"Good morning again Fatumata, sleep well?" Monique looked at me and smiled, addressing me in Bambara, and sat down at her rickety wooden desk facing the veranda.

Her question was the opening line in the traditional ritual of greetings. My choices of response were "Peace," "No problem," "Peace only," or "Really no problem." I assessed the night and decided to veer off the path and be honest.

"Hi, Monique, and no, I didn't."

I eased myself onto a green metal chair beside her.

"More wild dogs last night, eh?" She cocked her left eyebrow and chuckled. The idea that I was afraid of the semi-wild dogs that yipped and tussled nightly outside my window struck her as funny. (She had been far less mocking when a six-foot cobra had invaded my room, which a man had kindly removed and killed.) She also knew that my fear prevented me from braving the two-hundred-meter trek to the nearest nyegen to relieve a full bladder in the dark of night. Instead, I stayed safe inside and used a small bucket I had bought exclusively for that purpose.

"Yes, the dogs were outside again."

I looked at the examination slab in front of me, covered in pink stains from the medicine used to clean wounds and asked, "What happened to the boy?"

"He got his foot caught in the wheel of a bicycle, and he wouldn't let anyone touch it for days. It is seriously infected. I told his mother she must try and keep the foot clean and to bring him to me each day, so I can put on fresh wrappings."

Monique opened the trunk under her desk, pulled out her ledger and some individually wrapped pills, and began counting.

"What are those?"

"The small ones are aspirin," she said, "and these are Chloroquine. Do you have enough Chloroquine?" She held out a handful of the large white pills.

"Yes, the Peace Corps gives us bottles and bottles of it." So far, so healthy. The Paludrine and Chloroquine pills I flushed down my throat each morning had kept me malaria-symptom-free. Not malaria-free, as I, like everyone, had malaria in my blood just from being in southern Mali. The medicines were designed to keep the mosquito-borne parasites at a low enough level that one does not get the telltale symptoms of cyclic fever and flu-like chills and aches.

"Ah, *bon*," she said, putting the pills down on the desktop.

Time at last to bring up my small problem.

"But, Monique, there is something I need," I said, hoping I sounded less self-conscious than I felt.

"Yes?"

"I got my period. All my . . . feminine products are in my trunk that never arrived. So, I am wondering if you have anything I can use instead."

"Aspirin works very well."

"Huh? No, no, not the pain. I need something . . ." I glanced out the door in the unlikely event that someone who understood French was standing there. "Something for the blood. The products I need are, you know, made of cotton; you put them in your underwear . . ."

This was *so* embarrassing.

"Ah." She clicked her tongue in the back of her throat, to signal understanding, and nodded her head. "You put cotton in your underpants to absorb the blood?"

"Yes."

"We don't have that here. We use something else. Old pagnes."

"Old pagnes?"

She stood up and began to illustrate. "We take an old piece of cloth and we wrap it like this, and like this . . ." She moved her hands around her middle and through her legs, as if putting on an imaginary diaper. "And then we put on a pagne around us as usual, or maybe two if the period is heavy. We wash out the old pagne when we need to."

She stopped for a moment.

"Do you need some pagnes?"

"Ummm . . ." I thought a moment. Gym socks and bandanas suddenly seemed a breeze compared to the intricate wrapping of yards of cloth.

"No, I think what I have will do for now."

"You're sure, Fatumata? You also have aspirin, if you need it?"

"Yes, I do. Thank you."

She sat back down and began to write numbers in the ledger. Three blue-and-white beaded bracelets danced on her right wrist as she moved the blue Bic pen across the page.

With my mind somewhat at peace about the menstrual issue, it flooded with thoughts of the birth. It wasn't just the dogs that kept me from sleep. The previous night's experience in the birthing house had left me drained but exhilarated, my head dancing with the thrilling and terrifying images of life coming into the world.

"Monique, how long have you been the midwife here?"

"The dùgùtigi chose me, after the first year I lived here. I apprenticed with the *accoucheuses traditionelles*—traditional birth attendants—for two years. I attended many births with them, then did my nine months of health training, and became Nampossela's *matrone* and *aide soignante*— midwife and health worker. Little by little they have accepted me, and last year I started attending births on my own."

I already knew she had moved out to Nampossela from the larger town of Koutiala, as every woman moves to her husband's village, when she was eighteen. That was six years ago. I had no idea she had been on her own for only a year.

"Don't forget, tomorrow is baby-weighing day," she continued. "The world will be on my doorstep by this time in the morning."

"I'll be up early," I assured her. Tomorrow would consist of more than weighing babies. Women with young children from Nampossela and several neighboring towns walked here to talk about baby foods, weaning, and vaccinations.

"Well, who did the baby-weighing before you?"

"Nobody. It was not done."

"Nampossela is lucky to have you," I said. This was an understatement. Africa south of the Sahara, including Mali, has the fewest doctors and nurses per capita of anywhere on the globe. Nampossela was *extremely* lucky to have Monique.

Over the span of a hundred generations the village of Nampossela had literally been pulled from the ground, handful by handful, and shaped into mud brick homes and walls. Between these structures, paths had been beaten out by countless feet and hooves and washed bare by the force of the rains. These were not planned walkways so much as ways taken. A hot, shadeless walk along these paths took me every day from the guesthouse to Monique's in-laws' home in the heart of the village, the place where Monique cooked and did the domestic side of her seemingly endless work. This, not my castaway room in wild dog territory, was the place I had begun to think of as home.

Monique walked beside me, carrying a pile of branches on her head, Basil bobbing on her back. The branches stuck out at an array of angles, giving her a six-foot crown. She had positioned the firewood on top of a scarf, wrapped in the shape of a donut, and balanced it with one hand. She looked straight ahead to keep it level, her torso acted as a shock absorber, and each step she took, without glancing at her feet, was solid.

"We must plan your house," Monique said, as we turned right and entered an open space of a half-acre or so, near the middle of the village, the nearest thing to a town square in Nampossela. "Soon it will be time for the village to build you one."

"Where do you think I should build it? I'd like to be a little closer to town."

"The dùgùtigi will tell you. He knows the best spot."

The chief was a kind, soft-spoken man, who had taken me under his wing as soon as I arrived. Actually, he was one of two chiefs. Power was passed from father to son and brother to brother, based on age, along generations of Dembeles. The elderly Soungolo Dembele was the ceremonial chief but had transferred all his official power to Bakary Dembele, the man called dùgùtigi. As such, Bakary was recognized by the government administration as head of the village. He treated me as one of his own and called me daughter, *denmùso* (child-woman).

"I'm glad to know he'll help me," I said.

"He will. He has always helped me. You know, without him, I wouldn't have this work. Without him, Djeneba would still be Nampossela's midwife."

"Who is Djeneba?"

"You have not met her? The old midwife, short, with gray hair?"

"No."

"Ah, you will meet her one day, as she still helps me with the births. Remember when I told you that I apprenticed with the traditional birth attendants? Well, Djeneba Dembele was one of them. She and Helen Dao were getting old and the village wanted a third, younger midwife to help them."

We walked by the mosque, over twice as high as any other building in the village, made entirely of wood and mud. Most people in Mali, and in Nampossela, were Muslim. The call to prayer heralded the morning hour, a cascading, high-pitched summons, piercing the still dark air, and five daily prayers and washings measured the day. Facing the mosque was the small Catholic church where Monique attended services—a one-story, cement-coated building with a simple welded cross at the peak of its tin roof. About one in ten of the villagers were Christian, a high proportion for a Malian community. Behind the church, another religious tradition was represented by a miniature hut—home to one of the village's numerous fétiches.

Les fétiches (fetishes) were ritual objects used in the local Minianka religion, part of a complex system of beliefs and practices that protected the village and its people, regulated social interactions, and always had. Monique referred to the practice as *l'animisme* (animism). Whereas Islam and Christianity had found their way to the Minianka people, this religion had its beginning right here. Its followers worship *Klé*, the Supreme Being, through intermediaries such as fétiches and the spirits that are everywhere, in the water, the air, the earth, the animals, and in us. They had many special societies, mostly made up of men, who made animal sacrifices to their fétiches. Those who made the sacrifices were called *jŏ sonnaw* (fetish waterers), in Bambara or *féticheurs* in French. Even the Muslims and Christians were known to sacrifice chickens every now and then, wear protective amulets, use special potions and salves, or participate in various dances, funerals, and celebrations throughout the year. Everyone coexisted peacefully, for they were Minianka people first and foremost.

Past the church now, Monique and I entered a series of tighter passages, some lined with granaries, little round silos with thatched roofs. Monique had to walk carefully to keep her halo of branches from knocking against the walls.

"Ha! Here is a story for you, Fatumata. Years ago, when I was first chosen to be midwife, I almost died."

"What?"

"Yes, I became very sick with yellow fever. The people of the village, they said that it was the husband of Djeneba who put a curse on me. They said he was so jealous that I had stolen this position from his wife that he tried to kill me with poisoned words."

"How scary," I said, a cool tingle shooting up my spine. "Do you believe he caused the yellow fever?"

She laughed. "No, no. I told them, 'If I die, do not say that it was Djeneba's husband who killed me. If I die, it is God alone who has claimed me. Not anyone else.'"

After a few more turns, we entered the Dembele compound. The dirt yard, about the size of a large backyard swimming pool, was littered with rocks, big wooden mortars and pestles, piles of firewood, and blackened aluminum cooking pots waiting to be scoured. A small collapsed silo sat in a heap by the entrance and a family of goats fervently searched the ruins for grains of millet.

Three huts enclosed the yard, one for Monique's mother-in-law, Blanche, and sister-in-law, Elise, one for the family patriarch, Louis, and one for cooking. Monique, Basil, and her husband slept elsewhere, but I didn't know where. Monique's three-year-old daughter, Geneviève, did not live here at all but with Monique's parents in the larger town of Kou-tiala. (It was common practice for extended family to raise children, and though it was usually paternal grandparents who were in this role, Monique's mother was quite fond of Geneviève and did not want her growing up in a village where there was no school.) The women's and Louis' huts were rectangular two-room structures, each with only one door made of roughly hewn lumber. A couple of tiny windows placed high against the roof provided little ventilation. Nobody spent much time inside these stuffy caves, except to sleep or escape the rain.

The cooking hut was one room with a large opening on one side and no door. Two fires were going, each ringed by three stones balancing a steam-ing pot. The uneven walls were black from smoke. Next to the kitchen stood the nyegen, enclosed by scandalously short walls in dire need of repair.

Blanche and Elise sat against the wall of the women's hut in a long cool shadow. They were peeling onions and dropping them into a small wooden mortar.

"*Aw ni su*—Good evening," Monique and I said.

"Aw ni su," Blanche responded. She got up from her *sigilan* (small wooden stool) and held it out to me as an offering. She turned her shy, ancient, face toward me, yet did not look me in the eyes—the latter, a sign of deference. She was like an old deer, swaybacked and bent, her body moving lightly and quietly.

I accepted. Blanche glided over to the cooking pots, found an even smaller wooden stool that was missing a leg, and sat down again. Monique went into the cooking hut.

"Elise, give me some onions to peel." I reached my hand out to her.

"Ohhhh," Blanche said, smiling at Elise. Her eyes twinkled in her long face, but she covered her mouth, self-conscious about her missing front teeth. She found it amusing when I wanted to help. They were so careful with me, believing that I either should not, or could not, perform ordinary household chores. Because neither Blanche nor Elise spoke French, getting to know them during this first month had been slow. "Give me some onions to peel," was as personal and expressive as I could get in Bambara.

Elise, a spitting image of Blanche, but with fewer wrinkles and more teeth, scooped a few small onions from a half gourd that served as a bowl and handed them to me along with the knife. Her movements were like her thoughts—slow, as if each action left her somewhat bewildered. The family was having a hard time marrying her off. And she had baggage—a child named Karamogo, conceived and born out of wedlock. He was a sickly baby about a year old, with a big head perched precariously on a wasted body. He sat on the ground beside Elise, flies feasting in the corners of his listless eyes and droopy mouth.

I took the knife, a hammered-out implement with a dull blade, hunkered down, and began peeling. I was careful to remove only the outermost layer of dry skin. Yesterday, a neighbor had entered the compound, seen my discarded peelings on the ground, grabbed them, shook them in the air, and said something forcefully in Minianka. Monique translated for me: "I can flavor an entire meal with what you have thrown away!"

"Fatumata, good evening," said a small, hoarse, gulping voice in heavily accented French. Louis, Monique's father-in-law, had emerged from his hut. As always, he stood at attention, hands at his sides, a formality he had acquired while serving the French in World War II. He was about sixty-five, but his diamond-shaped face looked much older. It was heavily lined, and with his pointed ears and nose he looked like a wizened elf. He always wore the same stocking cap and baggy outfit, the unofficial uniform of the *cèkòròba*, (old man). Louis had once been a respected hunter and féticheur, but he had given that up some time ago upon converting to Catholicism.

"Good evening, Louis." I got up and walked over to shake his outstretched hand. He placed his other hand on the forearm of his shaking hand (another sign of respect) and nodded.

"Have you passed the day in peace?" he asked.

"Peace only. And how are you doing?

"No problems."

"*I Dembele*—You Dembele," I concluded, emphatically. I was honoring his family name.

"*I fana, i Dembele*—You also, you Dembele," he said.

He sat down on the end of a chaise lounge made of wood strapped together with dried sinews, and rested his gnarled hands on his knees.

I returned to my task. After a few minutes of peeling in silence I heard the sound of approaching static. A thin man with large almond eyes and tight lips sauntered into the compound, carrying a radio that was in desperate need of a clear station and new batteries. It was *le gars* (the guy), as Monique called him. I had barely spoken a word to Monique's husband and had only recently come to know his name: François. The guy wasn't around much, and when he was, there was unease between them. Monique spoke French, the guy did not; Monique had been to school, the guy had not; Monique was from Koutiala, and the guy was from this little village. I had the distinct impression that Monique had married down.

Tonight, the guy was dressed in jeans and a denim jacket with the collar turned up, Elvis-style. He didn't bother greeting us but sat down next to Louis, enjoying or oblivious to the sputter of his radio. He waited for Monique to serve him. It was customary for the men to eat first; the women and children ate what was left. Soon enough, Monique came out of the cooking hut with bowls of tŏ, the sticky millet porridge that is the staple of the Malian village diet, and smaller bowls of mudfish sauce for dipping. She walked past me without looking up, her expression hardened and cool. She placed the bowls of food on the ground in front of the men, along with bowls of water for rinsing the hands, and gave the slightest curtsy. Louis responded with a small nod, while François did nothing.

Goats were roaming the compound, led by their incessantly sniffing snouts and quivering lips. One of the scavengers was taking advantage of Monique's absence to wander into the cooking hut.

Monique came hurtling across the yard, yelling, "Ooo! Ush! Ah! Ta!" and pounding her feet. The panicked billy goat hoofed a quick retreat and then stopped just as suddenly at the compound entrance as if nothing had happened.

"That beast, I will drive him out!" Monique said and returned to the kitchen. She lifted a large pot off the fire, holding the metal sides with her bare hands, and quickly put it on the ground as she grimaced from the heat or the weight or both. Serving up more steaming tŏ, she brought it out and placed it in front of me. I was not expected to eat the men's leftovers. As a guest, I got my own bowl, which every evening I refused to touch until Monique shared it with me.

Louis thanked Monique for the meal, signaling he was finished. François simply pushed his bowl away. Monique picked up the bowls and presented them to Blanche and Elise, then sat down next to me. It was past seven o'clock and this was the first time all day I had seen her relax. She leaned one elbow on her knee and rested her head on her hand for a moment. Her thick, hard fingers spread across a yielding cheek.

"Let's eat," she said, and we dug into the light green, gritty paste. Methodically yet ravenously, Monique bent over the bowl, making a cohesive ball of tŏ with her hand and dipping it in the gooey brown sauce. She nudged the oily chunks of mudfish toward my side of the bowl, but I carefully dodged them. I was determined to remain a vegetarian, and I was glad it meant she and the others could have my share of meat. Elise was giving small pieces of tŏ to Karamogo, who sat in her lap and sucked on the food with disinterest. Monique slid Basil off her back and rested him in her lap. The rotund little fellow began to holler so Monique leaned back and put him to her breast.

A few goats stealthily inched their way back toward the hut and began licking the ground where a few drops of sauce had fallen. Monique got up, grabbed a long stick with one hand and, holding Basil in her other arm, thwacked the biggest goat with an "Ush, ush!" They once again ran toward the entrance, but Monique drove them into the corner of the compound by the fallen silo.

As if cued by the goats' departure, François got up and followed Monique around the corner and out of sight. I could just hear a hushed and angry exchange in Minianka. I glanced down quickly as Monique returned and the sound of the static faded into the distance. She sat down with a sigh, shifted her weight, rearranged Basil, and recommenced eating. I had never heard them argue and, not knowing what to say, concentrated on rolling a ball of tŏ between my fingers.

"Ah, ah, ah," Monique shook her head.

I hesitated, and then asked, "What's wrong?"

"It is nothing. I mean, it is just something between le gars and me," she said, and then added emphatically, "As always."

She glanced toward Louis' hut. He had gone back inside, but she kept her eye on the open door. She lowered her voice.

"Fatumata, you must excuse me for talking to you this way, but I don't know what I am going to do about this marriage."

Her sentence hung in the air. We both stopped eating and sat, unmoving. I was surprised at the revelation, not because of what she had said—it wasn't hard to guess that her marriage was far from ideal—but simply that she had shared it with me. I was curious to know what had just transpired. I glanced at Monique. Her eyes were alive, despite her stillness.

Two goats wandered over and halted, hovering near our food. They lowered their heads and raked their long grayish-pink tongues across the ground, following the drips toward our sauce bowl. Monique dove at them and slapped the largest one on the hindquarters as it turned away.

"Do you know what I think?" Monique asked, settling back onto her stool.

I looked at her expectantly, wanting to know more about François, wanting to understand what was wrong between them, wanting her to blurt it all out before Louis reappeared. Monique narrowed her eyes and pointed her finger at me.

"I think that all goats are going to burn in hell."

2

WEIGHING BABIES AND EATING DOGS

LOW PLANTS STRETCHED OUT IN LONG ROWS. They were so green and bright, so positively eager to be stripped of their seed. But that did not make up for my inexperience. I peered into my hand basket to inspect my meager collection of chickpeas. After an hour of steady picking, they barely covered the bottom. But I was glad to help the dùgùtigi and his wife Mawa in the fields. Mawa was very pregnant and working more slowly than usual, so I figured that I could put my chipper energy to good use.

My back and legs ached. I tried picking on one knee and then the other. I took constant swigs from my canteen. Never again would I take a can of chickpeas for granted. Meanwhile, the dùgùtigi and Mawa moved farther and farther down the rows, never stopping even for a drink. They gracefully took the plants in one hand and culled chickpeas into their palms in effortless motions. In the time it had taken me to collect a few handfuls, the dùgùtigi had gathered a sizeable pile in the hem of his tunic. Now he rose and dumped them into Mawa's large basket. She brushed aside the top layer of peas and pulled out a large one. She handed it to him with a smile and a nod in my direction. A large grin crossed his unshaven face and partly toothless mouth. He adjusted his large wool cap.

"This is from Mawa," he said in French with a slight lisp. Despite his years and status, he always looked down when he spoke to me—that sign of respect that I was accorded, as disconcerting as it was. "These two chickpeas stuck together mean your first children will be twins."

I stopped picking. It was a four-leaf clover game, Mali style.

"Twins!" I exclaimed in mock horror. "Why, I don't even have a husband! Oh, my father will be so upset. He always says, 'marriage first, *then* children.'"

The dùgùtigi translated for Mawa and they fell into fits of laughter; Mawa giggling so hard that her little eyes squinted to nothing in her moon-shaped face. The joke became a siesta; the dùgùtigi and Mawa sat down.

This was already going far more smoothly than my last attempt at working in the fields. Last week, I'd picked cotton with the village women. Cotton was the major cash crop of Mali, thanks to the French, and every villager grew some. It was hard on the soil, depleting vital nutrients, and it was hard on the hands, as each individual tuft had to be pulled from a thorny sheath. Women gathered for two days each week to work in one of their families' fields. They formed a line thirty to forty women strong that stretched across the width of the field, amidst Minianka songs that gave strength and swigs of *dòlo* (millet beer) that gave cheer. These incentives were not enough to keep me from being the weak link in an otherwise flawless female harvest machine. And worse, I had my period again, and I prayed that I would not be picking cotton more than a few hours so I could return to my room in time to change the socks and bandana. When the dùgùtigi appeared on the scene to check the work, he casually told me that he had brought his salidaga with him, full of water, and I could use it at any time if I needed to wash myself. I worried that I had misunderstood the French, and asked him to explain. He restated kindly, yet more directly, that he knew that I had *mes règles* (monthly period) and that I might need to wash. He had come to help. As I flushed crimson, a distinct disadvantage of being white, I couldn't help but ask how he knew. With a face full of wrinkles and patience, he said I should remember that he was fifty years old and had two wives and several teenage daughters—he had simply recognized the smell.

"Dùgùtigi, when can we pick the place for my house?" I sat back on my heels, several chickpeas in hand.

"Soon. Very soon."

"Monique has shown me around and I've seen some places where I'd like to build it."

"Very well. We will walk the village together. I am glad that Monique . . ." he pronounced her name Ma-nee-kee ". . . is a good jàtigi—a good host—for you."

"She's a good midwife, too."

"Yes, she never tires and she laughs with everyone. But it is not always easy for her." He sighed and his expression turned serious. "Because of her young age, there are women who will not come to her to give birth. They think it is the old women who must do this work. Some say that Monique is young enough to be their daughter and they don't give birth with their daughters. But the truth is this: those who give birth with Monique find a baby, and those who do not sometimes lose a baby."

He clapped his hands together, and then held his pink palms skyward, showing emptiness.

"Already, the women who birth with her talk to other women, and these others go to see her too." A fervent tone rose in his usually mellow voice. "Soon everyone will come to the birthing house of Nampossela."

I looked down at his bare feet, flat on the ground before me. They were thick like bricks, dry, with deep cracks around the heel. Covered in cinnamon-colored dust, they appeared to be growing out of the earth itself. He started to move ahead again. Apparently, our break was finished. I preoccupied myself with the four-leaf clover game and eventually found what I was after.

"Mawa, Mawa!" I called, taking up my basket, still lightly filled, and sitting next to her. I placed the double pea in her palm.

"Yuh!" she exclaimed and clapped me playfully on the back.

"What is it?" the dùgùtigi asked, joining us. Mawa showed him. They both laughed again. I may have been a poor picker, but at least I could provide a few chuckles. The dùgùtigi's face grew thoughtful.

"Twins are rare here in Nampossela, Fatumata. And even when they have come, they have not both survived." He seemed to think this over as he rolled the double pea between his fingers before dropping it in the basket to join its sisters and brothers.

Monique opened her tin trunk and took out the scale, a round disk like a clock face, marked off in kilograms, with a steel ring to hang it from. The scale reminded me of something from a corner grocery store in my childhood, only this one had a sling rather than a tray dangling from it. I took it from her and stood on a chair to suspend it from a hook near the door-frame. I attached the newly washed cloth harness (a frightened babe had wet it last week) as Monique got out a packet of blank charts for new arrivals. A chart recorded a child's progress—or decline—in the first years of life. Mothers were gathering outside. It was time to begin weighing babies.

The first woman came up and gave us her child's chart, retrieving it out of a deep fold in her pagne as if by sleight of hand. The clinic did not have a filing cabinet, so it was the mother's responsibility to keep the chart. I took the thin little girl and put her in the sling.

"Seven and one-half kilograms." Less than seventeen pounds.

"And she is over one year old," Monique said as she unfolded the green tattered paper and recorded the weight on the graph according to the child's age.

The graph was divided into colored zones: green meant fine, yellow beware, and red severely malnourished. The color coding was intended to make the chart easy to interpret for people who were not literate, which meant everyone in town except Monique and a handful of men. I had quickly noticed a trend. Most of the really young babies were healthy, but after they turned a year old or so, many dipped into the yellow and red zones.

"She is in the yellow," Monique said to the mother in Bambara as I got the child out of the sling. "She has lost weight. Has she been sick?"

"Yes," the woman answered, and they began a dialogue in Minianka. Monique raised her voice a little as other women gathered in the doorway to listen in and learn, some coming inside to sit on the floor of the clinic and others standing just outside. Monique used her arms and hands when speaking, clearly but gently pushing her words toward her audience. She looked around and made eye contact with everyone. The mothers clicked their tongues against the back of their throats in understanding. When the impromptu lesson ended, another mother approached with her baby, and the rest of the group dispersed onto the porch, picking up their conversations where they'd left off.

"That woman is pregnant again, her ninth child," Monique explained to me in French as I weighed the next infant. "She stopped nursing her child when she realized she was pregnant."

"Why?" I took the squalling infant out of the sling and handed him back to his mother. "This one weighs eight kilos."

"Ten months old. Still in the green, but barely." Monique carefully marked the chart before answering my question. "It is believed that the milk becomes bad for the nursing baby when a new one is growing inside. So she weaned the child right away and put her on adult food. The girl has had diarrhea ever since. I told her and the other mothers about the importance of not weaning abruptly, and about the importance of putting more time between their pregnancies. These are very, very common problems here."

She reached behind her, where Basil nestled in his sling on her back, and patted his bottom and protruding pudgy leg.

"He is almost four months old, three years younger than his sister Geneviève. And I will wait again to have my next baby. I don't care what le gars says," she added, lowering her voice.

Did François want another baby already? If so, how would Monique prevent it? I did not get a chance to ask.

"I ni sogoma," came a sluggish voice. Monique's sister-in-law Elise appeared in the doorway. She had cut to the front of the line and now approached Monique. She walked so pigeon-toed that her big toes almost touched. Her hand was wrapped in a strip of pagne. Strapped to Elise's back was her son Karamogo, his emaciated face and thin hair edged in dirt.

Elise had cut her finger this morning with a knife. After Monique cleaned the wound and wrapped it in a sterile bandage she motioned for Elise to put Karamogo in the sling to be weighed. Elise shook her head no. Monique spoke to her in Minianka for some time, but I could tell from Elise's tone that she was adamant. Finally she mumbled a thanks and left. The next mother approached and handed me her little girl. I put the baby in the sling and watched the needle jiggle and settle.

"Elise is lazy," Monique said. "And stubborn. I even have a chart for him, which I keep here, so she doesn't have to remember it. Did you know that 'Karamogo' means 'teacher'? She believes the name alone will give him a long life. Part of her knows Karamogo is sick, but she doesn't want to be told there is anything wrong with her son. And as you see, when she came here she did not even know it was the morning to weigh babies."

I took the girl out of the sling and handed her back to her mother. Monique recorded her weight on the chart. Green. Fine. Vaccinations up to date too. Monique spoke with the mother for a while. I was still thinking about Karamogo.

"What can we do about Elise?" I asked, when Monique was finished. She sighed.

"I asked her to please come next week. I'll remind her and we'll see if she does."

Another mother came forward, bearing her infant.

The next day for baby weighing came, but not Elise. Monique and I had little time to dwell on her absence. The last woman of the day was someone I hadn't seen before. She took a small tightly bound bundle off her back, and I gasped as she unwrapped it to reveal her child. Skeletal, his eyes bulging from their sockets, he seemed barely alive but for the flush of fever. His scalp was almost bare, his hair the scraggly filaments of an old, old man. Around his gaunt neck dangled two *gri-gris* (personal fétiches) for protection against sickness-inducing evil spirits. The woman was not from Nampossela and had no chart. She said her child was two years old.

"Weigh him carefully, Fatumata," Monique said.

I picked up his body, as brittle and hollow as a worn shell, afraid he would crumble in my arms. I'd read that two out of five children die before their fifth birthday in Mali. Now I felt it.

"Five kilograms."

He made soft mewing sounds when I took him out of the sling, as if he would cry but could not spare the energy or the tears.

Monique spent a long time talking with the mother. I watched, switching my attention between Monique and the near-lifeless child. When the conversation was over, the mother gathered up her boy and began walking at a brisk pace toward the road. Monique stood still, watching her.

"What's wrong with him?" I asked.

"He has had many attacks of malaria over the past few months. It has caused severe anemia, and now diarrhea. He is also malnourished. The mother didn't know what to do. She had not heard about malaria prevention and drugs. I told her she must go now to the hospital in Koutiala. It is only their medicine that can help, but even then, I doubt he will survive. She has waited too long. I can do nothing. I don't have IVs. I don't have serum. These women must bring me their children before they get so sick, then I have ways of helping them."

Monique looked at me, and then back toward the mother, who was now hitching a ride on a donkey cart. It would be a slow journey, exposed to the merciless sun, but it would be easier than walking the twelve kilometers.

I unhooked the sling from the scale and we started to clean up. Through the open slats of the window that faced the village, I saw a rider on a moped approaching along the path. As the figure got closer, I could see it was François, wearing a new jacket despite the heat. He passed by the clinic without looking up and continued onto the main road.

"*Merci!*" Monique yelled out the window. "Thank you for stopping to see if I needed anything from Koutiala!" She watched him disappear down the road. "Ah, he is good for nothing," she spat. "He thinks only of himself. If I had known his character, Fatumata, I never would have agreed to marry him."

She picked up a short broom and bent over to clean the floor.

"You didn't know him before you married him?"

"No. I knew his eldest sister, Yvonne, the one who chose me to marry him."

"She *chose* you?"

"Yes." She swept in brisk, circular motions as she told the story. "Yvonne was a kindergarten teacher at the school of the Catholic church in Koutiala. She was kind to all her students, but particularly kind to one. She followed this student very closely and took a great interest in her. One day at the inauguration of the church, she showed this girl to her younger brother and asked him to accept her for his future wife. That girl was me." Monique straightened and shook her head. "Yvonne and I always joked together and our families were good friends. I never had any problems with her. I thought it would be the same with him."

The broom rested idle in her hand. I tried to imagine what it would be like to know who my husband would be from the age of five. At twenty-two, I still had absolutely no intention of marrying.

As if she were reading my mind, Monique suddenly switched subjects.

"So, Fatumata, when do we get to meet Bakary Keita? He has yet to eat with us."

Bakary Keita was the Malian name of a fellow volunteer named John Bidwell. We had met during our Peace Corps training and had begun to get romantically involved. Our relationship had waned since I'd come to Nampossela, as he was assigned to a village on the other side of Mali. John was handsome and artistic, with a frisky sense of humor I found very appealing. I was interested and attracted, but torn. I had not come to Africa to start a long-distance relationship with an American. I'd already started pulling away. Playing this out would make things more complicated. What I did not tell Monique was that I was supposed to be seeing John at that very moment. Before leaving training for our respective villages we'd agreed to meet in Bamako for an embassy function. I was not ready to leave the village. There was no way to get word to John in time. He would now be in Bamako, but he would manage. I wasn't happy about leaving him in the lurch, but the decision to stay seemed right.

"He's planning to visit soon." Little did I know how soon.

"Very good. I am looking forward to meeting him."

I smiled, wondering what the villagers would think of him. In this southern region of short, dark men and women, John was a curiosity: six feet tall, blond, and blue-eyed. Young children sometimes screamed in terror on first seeing him, and older kids went so far as to stealthily pluck the exotic yellow hairs from his head.

Across the dry flat land dotted with dainty small-leafed neem trees, a small white pickup truck turned off the road François had taken and headed toward us. Its wheels churned up billows of dust. In a land of donkey carts and bicycles, a car was a rarity, a massive metal beast from another world.

Two men got out, clad in the crisp brown uniforms typical of *fonctionnaires* (government workers): slacks and an open-necked short-sleeved shirt with suit-jacket-style collars. Their shoes caught the sun despite a thin covering of red earth.

I recognized the driver, a small, thin man, as a member of the *Compagnie Malienne de Développement du Textile*, or CMDT, the largest Malian government agency in the region. I'd met the driver at their main office in Koutiala before arriving in Nampossela. CMDT's primary work was the cotton harvest—the village's main cash crop. Its agents were held in esteem, and slightly feared. They were responsible for weighing the cotton and providing the sole source of income for many villagers.

"I think that one is the Big Boss," Monique said in a whisper. She nodded at the stockier of the two as she put her broom down and dusted off her pagne.

The driver came forward, indicating the other man with a small wave of his upturned palm, a deferential flourish, before stepping to the side.

"This is Monsieur Diarra. He wishes to welcome you to the Koutiala region." Mr. Diarra took two majestic steps forward. I fortified myself for an exchange of formal greetings. I was barely able to perform this custom at normal speed in Bambara, let alone with sufficient fluency to impress the likes of Mr. Diarra. Then something about him struck me: his last name.

In Mali, *jàmus* (last names) were important because they defined one's lineage, which in turn, helped to determine one's place within the community. As a Dembele, the Diarras were my "joking cousins," a custom that dictated good-natured teasing between our families. Centuries ago, joking cousins were actually warring clans, but now the old hostilities had watered down to jokes and tame insults. These tended to run on well-worn tracks. A common jibe was calling someone a "bean-eater," implying that the person suffered from gastrointestinal distress. The Malian equivalent of a fart joke. "Dog-eater" was also an acceptable insult, a reference to the féticheurs and their followers, whose practice of animal sacrifice was looked down on by certain Muslims and Christians. In Minianka culture, dog sacrifice was particularly prevalent, making this insult a popular choice.

As a Dembele, my joking cousins included the Koulibalys, the Konés, and, as luck would have it, the Diarras. I could show off my cultural prowess.

"How are you?" I started.

"No problem."

I noticed out of the corner of my eye that two village women had shown up on the clinic porch, undoubtedly to see Monique. They paused and listened.

"How's your wife?"

"Really no problem."

"How's your dog?"

Silence.

"Have you eaten it yet?"

Pause.

"No problem!" he stuttered, and coughed.

Monique moved her hand across her face as if wiping off an offending substance, looked up at me, and smiled. It was a forced, fake smile. Mr. Diarra grew the same pained look. The two women snickered. I suddenly had a sinking feeling in my stomach. Had I confused the joking cousins' ritual? Mr. Diarra quickly regained his composure and the two men rambled through some pleasantries before saying their good-byes. The truck rumbled off, leaving a hanging trail of dust behind it.

I busied myself putting supplies away as Monique spoke with the two women who had come for antimalarial medicine. Once we'd exchanged the ritual good-byes with them, I turned to Monique, longing to find out what I'd done wrong in the exchange with Mr. Diarra. But before I could say a word, I heard someone outside the clinic door call my name. What now? I turned and saw it was Elise.

She stepped inside and asked Monique a question in Minianka. Monique gave a quick response and shook her head. Then Elise walked over to me, flicked her index finger to where my bra strap lay under my shirt, and pointed to her chest. I didn't need an interpreter. She wanted my bra. This request was not surprising. Bras were a luxury and few village women could afford one. Those who could, let their blouses slip and showed their straps with pride.

"Fatumata," Monique said in French, "I have an idea."

She turned to Elise. I caught a few words, "Karamogo," "healthy," and "*brassière*" among them. Elise's reaction was just north of ennui, but she began to take Karamogo off her back. I hooked the sling back on the scale and weighed him. He fell solidly in the red, but I could feel he had more flesh on him than the previous sick child. There was still hope.

Monique talked a long while with Elise, who stared at the colored chart with an amazed expression. I wondered if she could see, in its colors and lines, her child barely clinging to life.

As Elise placed Karamogo on her back, Monique turned to me and said, in French, "As you have seen, really all she wishes for is a bra. So, I told her if she comes every week to weigh Karamogo, she can have one."

What a great idea! It just might get her into the habit of caring for him.

Elise was barely gone before Monique burst out laughing.

"Oh, Fatumata! I must ask you something," she said, wagging her index finger and flashing her dark eyes, "Do you know . . .? Do you know what you asked Mr. Big Boss?"

"Yes, yes, I do. At least I think I do."

"You are very good at greeting people. You asked Mr. Big Boss how his family was, how his wife was, that was all fine. But then . . . I don't know quite how to tell you this . . ."

She bent over and giggled, then composed herself. Oh my, what had I done?

"Well, it is a very small thing. In Bambara, when you speak of something that is yours, you always put *ka* in front of the word, like when you say 'your house,' *i ka so*. But when you speak of a part of the body that is yours, you leave the *ka* out, like 'your hand' is *i bolo*. Do you understand so far?"

"Yes," I nodded, remembering this from my language training.

"Well, 'your dog' in Bambara is '*i ka wùlu*.' But you forgot the *ka*, and then you pronounced it *wulu*, rather than *wùlu*."

I could barely detect a difference in tone.

"You asked him about a part of his body," she spoke softly, leaning closer, though no one was around, "You asked him how his . . . thing was. You know . . . his male thing . . . down there." She searched my face for understanding. Her closed lips quivered in an attempt to stifle laughter.

"What?!"

"And then," she went on, "then you asked him if he had . . . eaten it!"

Monique lost all composure. She doubled over, gasping with laughter. I was mortified; my face burned and my flesh tingled. As she came up for air, she grabbed my arm and held on, swinging it back and forth while she laughed. Finally, she noticed my shocked stare and her amusement sputtered to a stop.

"Ah, Fatumata," she said, patting my arm in reassurance and dabbing her eyes. "This is not serious. We all knew what you were *trying* to say. You may have embarrassed yourself, but you have offended no one."

John showed up two days later and was not happy. He'd waited in Bamako for a day before concluding that something horrible had happened to me.

He tried to convince the Peace Corps office of this, but they were not moved. No news was good news as far as they were concerned. He found a bus for Koutiala and spent the night at a seedy hotel before finding someone to give him a ride on the back of a moped to Nampossela. He looked crazed. His hair was every which way, and red dust covered his face. Though he was relieved to see I was healthy, my defense for not going was not well received.

I insisted he stay for a few days before leaving again. He agreed and made an instant splash. While his language skills were poor and his fair complexion startling to the village tots, he made up for it all with humor. On a tour of the village, he stood in the middle of a herd of cows and mooed. Then he mimicked the bleat of an ewe so well that lambs ran to him, only to be frustrated at the udderless creature they found. At dinner, he serenaded Monique to the tune of "Volaré," never getting beyond "Monique-y, wo-wo, Monique-y wo-wo-wo-wo."

When John left, I was surprised to find that I missed him. His stay had gone better than expected, and I was more confused than ever. I was getting worried that this could get complicated, the very thing I swore that I would avoid. I wondered if I could push this relationship in the direction of friendship.

It would be a long time before Monique let me forget my linguistic faux pas with Mr. Big Boss. As we stood with the dùgùtigi beneath a large néré, or locust bean, tree in the field beside the clinic, she suddenly grabbed my hand and laughed. I knew what she was thinking about. I ignored her and concentrated on the task at hand: finding the little plot of land on which to build my self-designed three-room hut. It would be about the size of a one-car garage, made of mud brick coated in cement, with a corrugated tin roof and a small concrete patio. I was thrilled.

"You can choose any place that pleases you. All the land belongs to me," the dùgùtigi said, touching his chest with his fingers. "In fact, *this* very place is good."

"Um, it's too far from the village," I said, not liking the idea of being on the edge of town, alone. "Can we look around?"

We walked.

"How about over here?" I asked, as we entered a large communal area. It was near the hub of activity in the center of the village. Perfect.

"Ah, no, no, this is where the pigs wallow," the dùgùtigi said, shaking his head.

"It is true, Fatumata, there are many pigs here, and the well water here is always dirty," Monique said, then added, "Besides, this is where the Konés live, your joking cousins. You would have to ask them if they have eaten their dogs."

I fired her a threatening look. She raised her eyebrows.

The dùgùtigi started walking again. Was he smiling? We passed a gathering of huts shaded by mango trees and came to an open space.

"How about here?" I asked.

"Ah, no. Too close to the sacred well." He pointed to a large well on the banks of a nearby stream. We walked over to it. It was huge. A circular, meter-high wall surrounded by a concrete skirt. It had to be the only well I'd seen in the village that was not just a gaping hole in the ground. A small bulge on the skirt was covered in dried blood and feathers. A place of sacrifice.

"Why is it sacred?" I asked.

"It is sacred because it is where our village began," the dùgùtigi said. "Nampossela means 'village of the cow.' It was founded when a Dembele man's cow stopped to drink in this sacred stream and then refused to budge. That was hundreds of years ago, maybe a thousand. And this well is on the exact spot."

We walked and walked, me choosing a place and the dùgùtigi explaining why such a location would not work. Finally we found ourselves under the same néré from which we had started. The dùgùtigi looked around and nodded.

"How about here?"

Monique nodded too.

"Yours will be the first house in Nampossela's newest *quartier*," he said.

Now I understood. This had been decided long ago. I looked across the long dusty field to the village. Vast lengths of fields stretched out on all the other sides, but for a small grove of trees some distance away. No neighbors, no well or pump. But it seemed to be part of a larger plan. It was close to the clinic; that was good. And there was this beautiful tree with its spread of thick, winding branches and tiny fern-like leaves offering a small oasis of shade.

"Okay, this place will be fine," I said to the dùgùtigi, who praised my choice.

In reality, it still felt like the outskirts of nowhere, and this thought made me realize how much Nampossela was becoming somewhere for me.

"Each quartier of the village will provide bricks for you," the dùgùtigi explained with a shy smile. "Then you must go into Koutiala to get wood beams and tin for the roof. I will help you arrange for a donkey cart to bring everything back to Nampossela. God willing, we will have your house built before the rains."

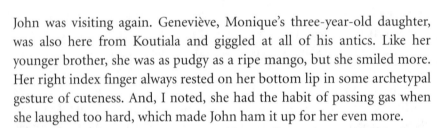

John was visiting again. Geneviève, Monique's three-year-old daughter, was also here from Koutiala and giggled at all of his antics. Like her younger brother, she was as pudgy as a ripe mango, but she smiled more. Her right index finger always rested on her bottom lip in some archetypal gesture of cuteness. And, I noted, she had the habit of passing gas when she laughed too hard, which made John ham it up for her even more.

"You both have the same sense of humor," Monique said, feigning a look of disapproval as she cleared away the dinner bowls. She wouldn't eat with me, now that John was here, insisting that he and I eat together. I'd have to work on that.

"Thanks for a wonderful meal, Monique," John said, leaning backwards and teetering on two legs of the stool.

"Fatumata and Bakary," came Louis' voice from his hut. He emerged and walked across the yard to us. "You must go into the village center. There is a *nya* coming through and entering its house tonight."

"What's a nya?" John turned to ask me.

"I'm not exactly sure," I said. "I saw a nya ceremony here before, when I visited for several days during our training. It was pretty wild, but I didn't ask many questions."

Louis came closer, standing straight as a pole as he spoke. His voice was always so relaxed, contrary to his posture.

"The nya is a fétiche that protects us. In Nampossela, there are many nya. A man will carry it on his back to its house, just over there." He indicated an area beyond the wall behind him.

"When he comes, you will see him, everyone will see him. He will jump and dance and turn, full of the power of the nya." Louis leaned over, one hand holding an invisible weight on his back, the other pretending to hold something ahead of him, and moved his dusty, bare feet in a quick rhythmic dance. John and I watched in stunned silence as he leapt, nimble as a child, into the air, his heels touching the backs of his legs before he again stamped the ground.

"If he touches anyone with the stick he holds, they will go crazy and die." Breathing hard, Louis settled into the reclining bamboo chair by the entrance to his hut to continue his explanation.

For many months, this nya had been in the forest. There, people made sacrifices of chickens and dogs, sometimes goats, bathing the fétiche in warm blood, imbuing it with life and power to heal their children and bring the rains that ensure bountiful harvests. After this "watering," and at the same time every year, this nya came home to the village, carried by a local man. The man visited the four quartiers, protecting them all, then walked through the center of the village, encircled the nya's small hut three times, and then placed the fétiche inside. There it would stay until the time came to take it back to the forest. Louis had once carried it, before receiving Christ as his savior.

It seemed the entire village was out to see the spectacle. John, Monique, and I elbowed our way along the paths jammed with excited people. *Balafons* (large xylophones) played over hollowed-out gourds, thrummed; *djembe* (hand drums) beat a hypnotic rhythm; people swayed; the air became tense and alive.

He entered from a nearby path, clad only in brown pants, a burlap sack bulging heavily against his back; inside was the fétiche. In front of him he held a thick stick over a meter long, attached to the sack by a cord. He dipped and swayed, staggered and flailed under the weight and almost visible power of the nya. His face was wet and his eyes rolled back into his head. As he approached, waving the stick wildly in the air, people either drew back to allow him to pass or fell and writhed on the ground before him. The three of us stepped back against a wall as he began to lurch in our direction.

He got closer and closer. The drumbeat quickened and shook the ground. The dust kicked up by the frenzied bodies clogged the air. Dozens of lanterns and torches cast a thousand shadows. Suddenly he was standing, hunched and quivering, in front of us. I tried not to flinch. His pole near our heads, I thought for an instant that he was going to crash it down on us, the unbelievers, the outsiders. Yet he whirled by and continued on, picking up speed until he was barely visible through the dust.

Able to move again, we drew away from the crowds and found the path toward the guesthouse. We strolled through the darkness, the noise and dust of the nya now behind us. After a minute, Monique broke the silence.

"Bakary," she said, "you haven't told me what kind of work you do in your village."

"Right now I'm mapping where all the wells and small dams are. Then we'll start repairing some of them."

"You repair wells in Sanso?"

"Yes. Open and eroded wells are dangerous . . . but you know that. I'm training men in the village to fix them. We'll cover the tops with concrete and put in a small door for pulling out water."

Monique nodded. Old open wells were indeed hazards. Debris dirtied the water. Children and animals fell in and were hurt or killed.

"Ba-ka-ry," Monique sing-songed. "We could use someone like you around here."

That night John and I walked around the perimeter of the village, my fingers intertwined with his. It was dark, the waning moon casting the weakest of light over the countryside.

"Nampossela is great, and Monique is a wonderful jàtigi."

In the distance huge white mounds emerged from the dark. The cotton harvest was almost over, and the millions of small tufts had been piled in four heaps, each the size of a house. Nampossela's *Association Villageoise*, or AV—an important group of village men, headed up by the dùgùtigi, who managed the funds and credit—had weighed each family's cotton. In truth, the cotton had been underweighed to avoid any errors and now it awaited transport by CMDT truck into Koutiala to be weighed once more. In addition to getting paid for the cotton, the village would then be paid the difference in these weights called *les accidents*, plus a 2 CFA (Communauté Financière Africaine francs: 1 CFA equaled roughly .002 cents) per kilogram *frais du marché* (cost of doing business), since the villagers weighed the cotton themselves rather than relying on CMDT to do it. If the village had any government loans or payments due for development projects, they would be taken out of this communal cotton money first. If the fund was not enough to cover these loans then the village was broke, and the loans had to be paid out of individual profits, a decision that could lead to many disagreements as the loss was distributed among families, sometimes not so evenly.

"Can you imagine playing in one of those heaps?" I said.

"Too much fun."

We paused for only a second before running over to the biggest pile and scrambling to the top. We jumped around, fell over, got cotton stuck in our hair, pulled it out, and did it all over again. John leaped into the air and spun. I took advantage of his imbalance and pushed him over. He rolled over on his back with a threatening stare, but before he could get up I fell on him. We sunk into the whiteness together.

I could not get accustomed to John being gone, to being the sole occupant of the guesthouse once again. With John there, I was not afraid to sleep outside on hot nights. In addition to the roaming packs of wild dogs, a "crazy woman," as the villagers called her, had simply appeared one day and stayed. They said that she was under the influence of an evil spirit, the victim of some terrible curse. Her hair was yellow and thick from the dust and she wore torn faded rags that barely covered her. She traipsed through the village at night, yelling in a language no one understood. By day she slept in an abandoned hut. This night promised to be especially hot and the guesthouse an uncomfortable, possibly unbearable place to sleep. I said so to Monique as we walked out of the compound after dinner.

"Tonight you can come to my house," Monique said. "Maybe you will sleep better outside with me, Basil, and the goats."

"I'd love to," I said, feeling a rush of relief.

I had yet to see Monique's house. She and François had a hut separate from Louis and Blanche's compound, but she did no cooking or eating there. In fact, she spent very little time at her own place, judging by how much time she spent at her in-laws', the maternity ward, and the clinic.

Our progress through the village was slow, as Monique chatted with everyone we passed. A few men sitting next to a glowing charcoal stove called us over to partake in their first round of tea. The nightly tea ritual took hours and consisted of three rounds of imported Chinese tea mixed with hefty quantities of sugar. The loose tea was boiled at great length in a small kettle, poured and mixed, and served up as greenish-black syrup with a caffeinated punch. We declined the offer politely, knowing the tea would chase any possibility of sleep away, and kept walking. I loved how the darkness faded the glare of my white skin; I blended in.

"Fatumata must get some *fru-frus*," Monique stated, as we approached a woman crouched beside a wide iron skillet. Balls of millet dough sizzled in bubbling oil. A few men on bicycles surrounded the woman, talking and taking fru-frus at will. I rarely saw anyone give her money. I asked for a dozen of the tangy, green, saucer-shaped treats. The cost was 50 CFA, about 10 cents. She lifted them from the oil with a slotted spoon, spread them on a ripped piece of notebook paper, and sprinkled them with sugar. I passed the parcel from palm to palm, blowing on the fru-frus until they cooled.

"Good evening, Fatumata," called a voice from the crowd. As a short woman approached, I saw it was Korotun. Thin and pretty in a severe way, she was a good friend of Monique, and the only one who spoke some French. She had a brusque manner about her and shamelessly asked me for things every time I saw her, mostly clothes and money. You never know what will fall from a tree unless you shake it, and Korotun kept shaking. I continually said no. I was not rich by Western standards (several pagnes, a short-wave radio, a small gas stove, a cassette player, a decent flashlight, a medical kit, and a forty-five-dollar-a-month stipend), but I had more than most villagers. And white people were synonymous with money, even in the dark.

"Good evening, Korotun," I said, Monique repeating the words right after me. I offered her some fru-frus.

"Fatumata," Korotun said, and reached out to hold my hand. "You must give me some money to buy sweet potatoes to fry up and sell. You know, some people think that I am rich, as I am married to Dramane," she said, eyes alight and lips tense, still grasping my hand. "The truth is, it is a rare day when he gives me money."

I knew Dramane. Just a few years older than I, he was the next Dembele in line to become the village chief. He was also a member of Nampossela's

Association Villageoise, and thus had access to village funds. The dùgùtigi had arranged for him to give me Bambara lessons, but he had only shown up for one and greeted me with half-lidded eyes that quickly glanced up and down my body. I remembered his coiffed and oiled hair, new jean clothes, and slight belly that shadowed his shiny belt buckle.

"Okay, Korotun. I'll lend you the money, and we'll work out a way for you to pay me back." This was better than a handout, and might give her some independence from her husband.

"Come, let Fatumata go, Koro," Monique said. "It is late and she is tired."

She pulled me away and we strolled on, following a path along a brick wall leading out of the village. It was indeed going to be a brutally hot night. Drops of perspiration rolled down my belly. The wall ended and we stood in a small clearing. To the right a few buildings were dribbled along the edge of the fields. To the left was a huge pile of cotton. It glowed white in the moonlight like a stranded cloud.

"I miss Bakary," I said, "I had such fun when he was here. And I think a lot about him when he's not."

"Then it is better that you stay with me at night. At the guesthouse, you will be alone in your own head. You will think too much."

"Very true. Monique, do you ever play in the cotton piles?"

"*Pati*—Oh my—no."

"Are they sacred, *ou bien*—or what?"

"No, no, it is just that they are not safe."

"How can playing in cotton not be safe?"

She cast me a skeptical eye. "Scorpions like to rest in them."

My jaw fell. Monique raised an eyebrow, and then stopped.

"*Voilà*. My great house," she said, pointing to the building closest to us. Ten yards in front of us stood a small rectangular box with a metal door. "As you see, there is no fence, no nyegen, and no cooking hut."

How could this be her home? She was the health worker and midwife, one of only a handful of people in the village with a paid job. Monique searched for the right key in the dark, and unlocked the door. There were two rooms. One held grains in large tan sacks, hanging baskets of spices, and piles of clothes draped over ropes slung between two posts. The other room had a large, straw-filled mattress on the dirt floor, several straw mats rolled into fat cylinders, two straw-filled pillows covered with red polyester, and a tin trunk. A kerosene lantern hung from a peg by the door.

Monique lit the lantern, picked up one of the pillows, and began dragging one of the mats outside. Several goats and a donkey approached, as if expecting to be fed, and stood right on the mat.

"Ush. Ush," Monique blurted, scattering the animals. "Here is where Fatumata will sleep well tonight." She put the mat on the ground, just to the left of the open tin door, against the front wall of the house. Then she dragged out another mat and pillow, placed them on the other side of the door, and sat down. She slung Basil off her back, swung her two legs to the side, and placed him between her ankles. He immediately let forth a long stream of pee.

"How did you know he had to go?" I asked, amazed.

"I know the body movements he makes when he has to go." She shook Basil's lower half and placed him on the mat beside her. "If he had had to poop, and I didn't want to clean it up off the ground, I would use a little plastic pot," she said as she leaned back, reaching just inside the hut's front door, ". . . like this." She presented a small plastic bowl, the size of a cereal bowl, with a handle and a big round lip. There were no diapers here, and yet I hadn't seen women's clothes or backs wet and smeared with baby poop. A mother's attention and a small bowl did the trick. Miraculous.

"Ha!" Monique laughed as she lay down on the mat, Basil folded into her body. "The villagers have said there are bad spirits out tonight, that everyone must sleep inside with the doors and windows closed, or the spirits will drive them insane. They will be locked in their hot houses with the doors shut tight. We will see, huh? We will see who will be the crazy ones in the morning."

I looked down at my bed, then into the hut. It occurred to me that I was taking François' pillow.

"Is it okay with le gars if I sleep here?"

"Le gars? He will not be coming home tonight. There is someone visiting him. He ate his meal elsewhere in the village and will sleep there as well. With her."

"Oh." I gulped. "You are not upset?"

"What can I do?"

Mother and child yawned loudly, in unison. I lay down too, but every time I shifted positions on the hard ground, the straw mat crunched. I was not used to the absence of bedtime ritual. No changing clothes, brushing teeth, or reading a book, no sheet to cover and protect me.

I stared out toward the fields. Monique's home was built on the edge of Nampossela, just like mine would be. The animals came closer, sniffed me, and settled down. Apparently they did not like being alone any more than I did. A couple of goats nestled against the wall by my head. The donkey stood close by, filling the night with the slow swoosh of its grassy, sour breath. I tuned my senses to the approach of evil spirits, whatever they might sound or look like, but my awareness only magnified the small movement of hooves and moist ruminating mouths. I imagined this land before people and their domesticated animals tamed it, when it belonged to the wild beasts: the lions, hyenas, elephants, and hippos. I looked up, past the animals, over the huts, straight up into the star-packed night, wide-awake and thankful to have escaped the confines of the guesthouse. Thankful to be here, with Monique, under a vast and dizzying sky.

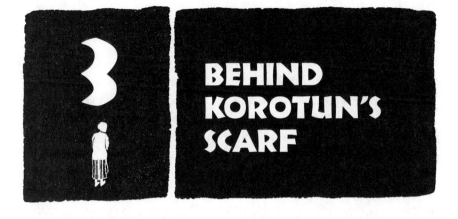

3

BEHIND KOROTUN'S SCARF

IT WAS THE BEGINNING OF THE DRY SEASON. The season for building. Bricks were molded and dried in the sun in long rows, looking like hundreds of miniature subdivisions. The villagers used them by the thousands to rebuild walls and silos and, this year, to build my house. I watched it arrive in slow procession via donkey cart, brick by brick, as I leaned back against the wall of the dùgùtigi's abandoned home.

Monique arrived at the clinic later than usual and walked out.

"Good morning, Fatumata."

"Good morning," I said. "Where have you been?"

"At the birthing house," she said as she cleaned her teeth with the frayed end of a neem tree branch, the equivalent of a toothbrush here.

She stretched and yawned, lowered the small branch, then cupped the left side of her mouth.

"Oh, the pain in my teeth is killing me today."

"What's happened to them?"

"Nothing. I have holes on the left side. It is getting so bad, I will soon have to chew with the other side only."

"There are no dentists, no teeth doctors here?" I doubted it, judging by the decayed state of the teeth I had seen.

"Teeth doctors? No, no. I have heard of them. But they are in Bamako."

Basil was wide-awake on Monique's back, and uncharacteristically quiet. He stared at me with big eyes and even seemed to grin a little. That was new.

"I have some good news for you," she said with a smile. "The dùgùtigi's wife, Mawa, has given birth."

"When? The birth was this morning?"

"Yes. She labored all night and gave birth today."

Her smile opened into a wide yawn.

"And Mawa is okay? And the baby is okay?"

"Yes, they are doing fine. The dùgùtigi is on his way himself to inform you."

Minutes later, the dùgùtigi came walking through the field toward us, he stopped a moment to look at the bricks atop a donkey cart, and then greeted us.

His lined face beamed. Grins were infectious today.

"Daughter, I want to tell you my news. Mawa gave birth this morning."

"Congratulations. I'm so happy for you. How is Mawa? How is the baby?"

His smile broadened. So did Monique's. Even Basil grinned. This was getting absurd.

"Mawa is in good health. The babies are also in good health."

"Babies?!"

"Yes, twin boys."

The chickpea prophecy had come true.

"Yes, the birth was difficult, but Monique was there. We thank God they are all fine. We thank God I have two sons." He took a deep, happy breath and continued, "I have made a sacrifice of two white chickens. Two white chickens in your honor."

I pictured him squatting over the sacrificial stone near the old well, stretching wide the neck of a struggling bird, white feathers floating on the wind, his knife spilling life's blood as protection for his sons.

"*Allah k'aw bolo. Allah k'aw kisi banaw ma.*" I said, benedictions for a healthy life, free of sickness.

The sun had set, but the oppressive heat of the day persisted. The moon showed only a fingernail of light, giving no illumination to the rough path through the village. Monique and I walked by flashlight to our friend Korotun's compound. I was eager to find out if the fried sweet potato business that I had helped her set up was turning a profit. But first, Monique had an important errand to do with another family.

"Adama must let Natou rest," Monique said with a touch of exasperation, as we headed deep into the Dembele quartier. "He has two wives. He can let the other one do Natou's work for a while."

Adama Dembele held the important post of secretary and treasurer in Nampossela's Association Villageoise. Only in his late twenties, he was young for such a position. This was in large part because he was a Dembele and the dùgùtigi's cousin, and he could read and write. Natou was Adama's first wife.

Natou had given birth to their third child two days before. Just yesterday one of Natou's children had raced into Monique's compound and blurted between heavy breaths that Natou had fainted and was bleeding. It was common for a woman to put in a full day's work soon after giving birth—pounding millet, washing clothes, hauling water, cooking over a hot fire, and sweeping out the compound—but usually they were allowed to rest for at least a week. Monique believed they should be allowed to rest and not participate in heavy lifting longer than that.

After stopping Natou's blood flow, Monique laid out a mat in Natou's hut and admonished her to rest, with her feet up, for a day or two. Monique explained to the new mother that she was at risk for more bleeding. She had endured a difficult labor and was lacking iron. When Natou complained that there was too much work to be done to rest, Monique told her that now was the time to rely on the work of her co-wife. Finally, Natou nodded her consent.

But despite these warnings, just this afternoon Monique had caught Natou returning from a well with a twenty-liter basin of water teetering on her head. So now it was necessary to talk with Adama. As the husband, he made the rules of the house. If Natou was going to rest and heal, it was Adama who ultimately needed convincing.

"He is the father of four children," Monique said." I have talked to him about the dangers of women carrying heavy loads before."

"So, what do you say this time?" I asked.

"Ah, I must be aware of what comes out of my mouth. A woman's husband must always be handled with care, especially this one."

Monique had to make sure that her instructions were followed without Adama losing face. Just as important, she had to avoid angering him. He was responsible for paying her salary.

As we turned to enter his compound, we almost bumped into Adama coming out.

"Ah, *I ni su*," Monique said, giving the evening greeting.

"I ni su," Adama said to Monique and then to me, "I ni su, Fatumata." He continued past us without pausing. Off one shoulder hung a small backpack. With my flashlight I could just make out the words Chuck E. Cheese written across it. First a child's book bag, now a symbol of status. He held a deck of cards in his swinging left hand.

It was *belotte* time for the elite of Nampossela—the young men whose minimal schooling or family connections allowed them to attain paid positions in the village hierarchy. Access to money and less reliance on farming gave them leisure time to indulge in belotte, a popular card game. Almost every evening, four or five of them could be found sitting around a small wooden table in the center of the village. They gambled far into the night, leaning back in their chairs, cigarettes dangling, dirty coinage piling up, surrounded by a rotating entourage of young female admirers.

"Adama," Monique called, "I'd like to speak with you for a moment."

Adama stopped, turned, and faced us. He was a rather severe-looking man, with a long straight nose, lips that naturally turned down, and an erect carriage that made him look taller than he was. Like other important young men in the village, he preferred Western-style clothes: a button-down shirt and tailored polyester pants.

"Yes. What is it?" Adama asked impatiently.

"It is about your wife, Natou," Monique said, walking past me and drawing nearer to him." She needs to rest for the next four days, until your son is named. I have told her this and now I am telling you."

Being Muslim, Adama's family would name the baby on the seventh day after birth. Adama gave a brief nod and brusquely turned to walk away again.

"Adama," Monique called, "I am almost finished."

I felt that Monique was pushing it.

"Adama, you are a good Muslim, and a good husband," Monique continued. "You know Natou had a very long labor. She is tired from it. I told her that she must not carry water for two weeks. Now I am telling you this because I know you understand. Your son will not be healthy if his mother is not. That is all. May God protect them."

"Amen," Adama muttered, giving Monique a hard gaze as he turned to go. Monique looked after him, and then let out her breath in a short sigh.

"Now," she said, turning back the way we had come, "to buy some millet fru-frus to take to Koro. She is too skinny these days."

Korotun and Dramane were wealthy by village standards. Their house had a tin roof rather than one of mud and branch, and a small concrete patio. Welded iron chairs with plastic woven seats (called *fonctionnaire* chairs, after the government workers who could afford them), not wooden stools, were arranged in a rough circle around a small charcoal burner. A tiny blue teapot, hinged lid open, sat astride the cool black coals.

"I ni su," Monique called. The door to the house was open. A faded, almost translucent curtain hung across it, glowing amber from a lantern inside and providing the only sign of warmth in the compound.

"I ni su," we heard from the hut, barely audible, but unmistakably Korotun's husky, direct voice.

"Sit down Fatumata, let's wait for her," Monique said.

As I sat down in a chair, Korotun's slim outline broke through the thin membrane stretched across the doorway. She shuffled out, carrying the lantern in one hand, while her other hand cloaked one side of her face with her headscarf.

We exchanged brief greetings as she slumped into a chair next to Monique.

I offered up the plastic bag of fru-frus. She looked emaciated: her collarbones formed steep ridges under her red blouse. As she reached for the bag the scarf fell away from her face. The lantern light was dim, but I could see that one side was swollen, her eye half closed with puffy tissue. She met my stare, lowered her gaze, and quickly draped the scarf back over.

We sat in silence. The heat of the earth radiated up, drying my throat and nose. I felt heavy.

"Ehh, Koro . . . puh, puh, puh," Monique said. "What happened?" Her voice was gentle, but firm. A thin line of anger edged her tone.

I stared at the ground, not knowing what to say or do.

Korotun whisked off the scarf and looked at us dead on, giving us a full view of the damage. "So you see, you see his work. The work that he has done to me tonight." Her voice was high and sputtering, "This face is not all. No. Here. Here, look at this." She thrust her right arm out and lifted the sleeve. Across her upper arm were striped welts, the engorged and painful shadows of her husband's fingers used as a vice.

"I can barely move this arm, it hurts so much." Korotun spit out the words into the night. "I think I am leaving. I am packing up my things and going back to my village."

Monique glanced at me.

"Korotun, I can understand if you want to go. Maybe that would be the best," she said, and then thrust her arms into the air, as if freeing something from her chest. "How many times have I spoken to him and said to work it out? Try and not bother each other and work it out. But Dramane, it is his way. Always he has been like this. But this time . . . what happened?"

She looked at Korotun and grew still.

"Ah, it is like this . . ." Korotun paused, and then unleashed a stream of words. "Dramane came home drunk tonight and did not find me here, at home. I was in the middle of town, selling sweet potatoes, making us some money. But when he found me, did he thank me for this? No! He dragged me back here, screaming that I was out to walk the village and flirt with the men. And then . . ." Her fingers hovered over her face, hesitant to touch its new topography.

Monique moved closer to Korotun and began examining the cuts and bruises on Korotun's face with the flashlight, and gingerly testing her arm. Korotun winced, but made not a sound.

"Koro, I must dress the side of your face. Your arm will be very sore for a while, but it is not broken."

"What am I supposed to do? How am I to cook? How am I to peel my millet? How am I to draw water? Huh? Huh? With this alone?" She raised her unhurt arm in the air and looked fiercely at me, her one good eye alert and filled with desperation.

"Fatumata, you must help me."

"I . . . how . . . What can I do?" I said, thinking that I had already helped enough. She would not have had the money to buy sweet potatoes had it not been for me. As I looked at her bruises, I thought about applying ice. Not a realistic option.

"Get me some medicine so I can have a baby, so Dramane will not get so angry. He thinks I take something so that I will not get pregnant, so I can sleep with other men, but this is not true. You must know of something to make me pregnant."

"I don't really know of any medicine that will make you pregnant. There are vitamins you can take to make you healthier so you'll be more likely to get pregnant, and there are medicines to treat diseases or infections that may be preventing you from getting pregnant . . ."

"Yes, the vitamins. That's it. That's what I need."

"We can find those at the pharmacy in Koutiala," Monique said quickly, deflecting Korotun's next question, which would surely entail asking me for the money. "I can get you some."

"Okay, I will try that," Korotun said to herself more than to us. "I will tell him I am on medicine that will get me pregnant. I am on Fatumata's medicine."

I kept my mouth shut. None of this had been covered in my Peace Corps cultural training. I wondered if her infertility had anything to do with her thinness. And whether that had anything to do with the stress of living with Dramane.

"For now, I must get medicines to tend to your face." Monique said, closing the conversation. "I'll be back."

Not wanting to stay and be asked for more things, I accompanied Monique out of the desolate compound to retrieve supplies. The paths were lined by weathered brown walls, all of them made up of the backsides of families' huts and compounds. There must be other women like Korotun, trapped and hurt behind these walls.

"Monique, is Dramane beating Korotun just because she can't get pregnant?"

"Ah, Dramane *le bandit*. Le bandit who thinks he is a king. Yes, because he wants a child, because he is a jealous man, because he drinks too much. But what good will beating do? Eh? Some men believe that their wives must be 'educated' in this way. It is not okay."

"Why doesn't she just leave him?"

"That would not be easy for her. She chose to marry Dramane, though her family did not wish it. They will not hear her cries for help."

So Korotun's marriage, her *furu*, was her choice and not her family's. I knew the Minianka were patrilineal, where the woman becomes part of the husband's family, and children carry on their father's name and ancestral history of taboos and fétiches. How the system worked when the families hadn't agreed to the union, I didn't know. But I imagined that the benefits of an arranged marriage, the investment of the families to work out problems and build relationships, were not hers to enjoy. She was alone with her decision.

We turned off the path and followed a long wall. Monique fell into her own thoughts. A cicada's deafening chirp filled the air.

"Ha! If ever, if ever le gars tried to hit me . . ." she mimed a slap, "God would not want to see what I would do."

"François hasn't ever hit you?"

"Never. We argue, but he is too afraid of me to hit me."

"I'm glad to know he doesn't hit you," I said. "You know, men hit women in my country too."

"What? You are joking!"

"Yes. In the United States it is a big problem." I said. How to explain the isolation of our nuclear families, living apart from extended family and old friends? The women, like Korotun, with nowhere to go? I saw the concern in Monique's eyes, and qualified my statement with "Not all the men do it, I don't mean that. But some do, and the women don't know how, or are too afraid, to get help."

"Oh, this is very serious. Then it is the same problem everywhere," she said. "But I think that Bakary would never do that to you."

"No he wouldn't," I agreed. "Besides, he is too afraid of me to hit me."

I looked at her to see if my attempt to lighten the atmosphere had registered, but she just nodded her head.

In the weeks that followed, I could not rid my eyes of the image of Korotun's beaten face. Even as her skin healed and smoothed, the injuries bumped and jostled my thoughts. They even seemed to mark a shift in the weather. Ever since Korotun's fallen scarf had given me a glimpse into her turbulent world, the dry harmattan winds had begun to blow hard from the north. The sky became reddish brown with topsoil, and dust devils roamed the fields, spiraling dead leaves, husks, and stray plastic bags into the air. Every time the sky turned overcast, villagers rushed to close windows and doors and protect food, clothes, and eyes from the rainless storms of advancing dust. Undeterred, grit slid into every crack, slipped under every door, filled every body crease.

The earth had gone five months without a drink, and it would have to wait another four before the rains began. Life was ruled by the need for water. Water for drinking, water for cooking, water for cleaning. Dragged from the bottoms of shallow wells, filled with sediment, sometimes disease-ridden, it was rationed and almost worshipped. The only respite was an occasional freak shower, caused by a shift in air currents that brought up moist air from the coast. Light and short, it was just enough to be a reminder that water would be plentiful again.

And after the dry season came the hot season, as the humidity built up before the big, soaking rains. Though it was only February, the nights were distinctly hotter. It looked like my house would be completed before the rains, and I was thankful. The speed and skill with which the villagers were building it convinced Monique and I that they could tackle a bigger project: the birthing house.

With its ripped-up roof, termite-eaten beams, and rain-stained walls, the birthing house was a constant source of grief to Monique. "Women cannot stay here during the rainy season," she had complained more than once. It was built by the Chinese over a decade ago with the idea of harnessing the power of biogas to provide stove fuel and electric lights in the building. Biogas was generated by the *misibofuntenidinge* (cow dung heat hole), a small shack over a deep hole in the ground that was supposed to be filled with soupy manure. It had hardly been used and remained a curiosity.

Knowing it would cost too much money, Monique had never spoken with the dùgùtigi about repairing the building, despite the obvious need. But if the village could supply the bricks and labor, as they were doing for my house, I could find USAID (United States Agency for International Development) funding for the rest through a special fund they had for small Peace Corps projects.

It was too late to do the work this year, but Monique and I broached the subject one evening with the dùgùtigi. I explained to him that I could find money for two-thirds of the cost, if the village paid for the other third, most of which could be supplied in labor. At first, he wanted the money to be used to complete his roofless dream home, but understood when I explained that the money had to be used for community projects. If the village elders gave their consent, and we received the funds, it could be repaired next year.

"It is a matter of education, Fatumata. After our meeting today, the women will understand *konoboli*—diarrhea—and how to treat it."

Monique and I were walking to a neighboring town, N'tabugoro, eight kilometers away, to conduct a health meeting with women about sanitation and sickness. One key topic would be the importance of giving children fluids when they have konoboli, literally "stomach running."

"The mothers see that when they give their child water, it increases the konoboli," Monique explained. "While we know the water rehydrates, they see only that it gives more konoboli."

"I guess that makes a kind of sense," I said. "If you view the diarrhea as bad and see that giving no more water stops it, you stop giving the water."

We passed a hamlet nestled beside the road; it was a small compound surrounded by dusty fields. Monique said it was the home of an old family friend.

"Come," she said. "We still have a little time to visit. If someone tells them that I have been here and did not stop, I will never hear the end of it."

She introduced me to the ancient man and his wife. We sat and chatted. The elder man was a renowned féticheur and he offered to divine my future. Clad in the dark heavy weave of mudcloth, heavy strips of cotton cloth sewn together and dyed with mud, called *bogolanfini*, he sat in the shadowed heat of a closed hut and threw cowry shells in the sand. Through their arrangement he peered into time. He told me that I would have no enemies in Mali. He said a white man in Mali would ask me to marry him. But these things would come to pass only if I chewed a *yelewòro* (smiling kola nut)—so named because of the curved crease in its middle—on a Thursday. Kola nuts, known for the mild stimulant effect of their bitter yellow pulp, were an elder's prerogative, a substance that provided a little geriatric zest.

"Yuck, I can't stand the taste of those things," I said when we had rejoined the road to the village. "But it would be nice to have no enemies here."

"Ha! We will ask *every* old man to show us his pile of kola nuts," Monique said with a laugh. "We will find a yelewòro, so this prophecy of a husband comes true!"

Evidently she and I had taken different ideas from our encounter.

We then stopped by her Uncle Basil's house to give brief greetings. (She called him "father," as she did all her father's brothers. When I asked about this, she said that in the Minianka language, the words "aunt" and "uncle" don't exist, only "mother" and "father," but in French, she could say "uncle.") A Christian by name, and a féticheur by practice, Basil gave a pat to his namesake on Monique's back and dug through a number of kola nuts in his shirt pocket to find one that smiled. No luck. Finally, we arrived in the town center, where about twenty-five women and their assorted small offspring were waiting for us. Monique greeted everyone, introduced us both, and made the women laugh by pointing to my backpack filled with papers and a water bottle, and saying I, too, was a mother, and this was my son. It was a perfect way to warm up the crowd and put them at ease with this tall, childless white woman. I asked the women what they knew about diarrhea, its causes, and cures. A few women said that konoboli was caused by cold weather; another mentioned malaria, and another bad spirits. For cures, many mentioned traditional medicine, totems, and not giving food or drink.

Thus began our discussion of germs and prevention: the importance of drinking clean water, covering food from flies, and washing hands with soap. Monique talked at length about remedies and the difference between dirty, germ-ridden water that is harmful and can cause diarrhea, and clean water that helps the sick child get well. We showed them how to make keneya ji (health water), a mixture of salt, sugar, and clean water used for rehydration. We watched as a few women came forward to prepare some. Prepackaged oral rehydration mixes were available in pharmacies in Koutiala but were prohibitively expensive. Monique and I left the women with a few bags of sugar and salt to distribute among themselves and began the long walk back to Nampossela.

Upon arrival, Louis, with the help of a few of the elder Dembeles, located a yelewòro. His craggy fingers placed the eyeball-sized, yellow nut into the palm of my hand. The curved crack running along its length did indeed mimic a grin. I chewed its flesh and spit its orange, stringy carcass onto the earth as Monique sang in joyful noise about husbands, and I hoped the bitter experience was worth having no enemies here.

I was awakened late one night by cramps ebbing and flowing, by a force gathering in my bowels, a force that was preparing to exit my body from both ends. This posed a serious logistical dilemma. I would never reach the nyegen, two hundred yards away. I fumbled in the dark for my flashlight, and dragged my two plastic buckets toward me. I hitched up my sleeping dress and crouched over one, holding the other under my chin. The result was a sour, sulfury mess, but I didn't care. I fell onto the cool floor and passed out.

This cycle continued through the night until I wondered if I might expire from intestinal distress and olfactory overload. I had never felt so utterly alone. I knew I needed water. I crawled to the water jar just outside my room, in the antechamber. It was cool and I rested my face against it. A wave of panic swept through me as I realized how far away I was from the buckets, but it lasted only long enough for me to pass out again.

I awoke to a blinding sun banging at my door.

"Fatumata, Fatumata . . . are you in there?"

The sun sounded like Monique. Part of me knew this was not a dream. I opened my mouth, but could hardly make a noise.

"Monique," I croaked, "I'm sick."

She unlocked the antechamber door with her key.

"Oh my God, Fatumata. What happened? What happened?" I could just make out a dark form standing over me.

Hot tears came streaming down. My shame could not hide, even behind my sickness.

"Ah, ah, ah, it's okay, it's okay," she said as she ran her hand over my forehead and hair, pushing the damp curls back from my face. "I will make you some keneya ji."

Keneya ji, the rehydration drink that just days ago I had been showing others how to make. Monique quickly returned with her concoction in a clean drinking cup, and encouraged me to take small sips. She then went into my room, exclaimed "Pati!" and came out, tightly gripping the buckets. She took them outside and began to speak to those already in line for the clinic. The door creaked open and staring children appeared.

"Ush! Get out of here. Get out of here or I will beat you!" Monique entered the anteroom, pushing the kids aside.

"I have sent someone to bring you water," she said, "so you will be able to bathe. Let's rest you in your bed until she comes."

I got up on my elbows and, with Monique behind me, rose slowly to my feet. The explosive power of last night's trials was evident all over my dress. Hunched over Monique's steady body, I managed to get to my bed. I sank into my straw mattress, soft as a bed of clouds after a night on concrete. Using two sides of a cardboard box like a whiskbroom and pan, Monique cleaned up the puddles of diarrhea and vomit. Then she sprinkled sand over the floor, let it sit, and swept that up with a broom. I had seen this done before when mothers cleaned up after their babies.

"Never thought that you'd be cleaning up after me like Basil, did you?" I asked, feeling a little better with drink and company.

"Mali sicknesses are bad. And you are not used to them," Monique said.

Sicknesses. From what I had learned in training, this one seemed to be a bout of giardiasis. Caused by a parasite in the oral-fecal cycle, it resulted in violent, sulfur-smelling emissions.

Just then a voice outside called out in Minianka, "Fatumata, your water." I heard the crash of water cascading into the mouth of my clay jar in the antechamber. A waterfall of life. I could imagine it pouring from a basin balanced on some girl's head, and I was sure that not a drop was spilled. Water, precious water.

"Do you remember Oumou? Daouda's wife? The one with the son named Gwewa?" Monique asked. She came over and sat on the edge of the bed.

"Yes." The well digger's wife. I said hello to her frequently as I walked to Monique's. She was quite friendly and always surrounded by rambunctious children.

"Oumou came to me early this morning to give me the news that Gwewa died yesterday. He had diarrhea for days and days, and fever too. She made keneya ji for him, but it was too late. He did not recover."

Monique's jaw was set hard in her face. Little wonder children died so quickly. Their life force literally exploded from their bodies in a matter of hours. I deliberately took more sips. I was not merely drinking; I was keeping myself alive.

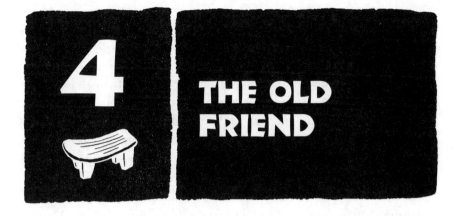

4

THE OLD FRIEND

"GOOD MORNING! YOUR COFFEE IS HERE," I CALLED, WALKING ONTO THE CLINIC VERANDA AND STANDING IN A COOL SPOT NOT YET TOUCHED BY THE RISING SUN. Two flies buzzed near the mugs I held in each hand, desperate to land on the rims. After my bout with giardiasis, I was all too aware of the intestinal havoc wrought by these evil germ-ridden insects. It had taken days before I could eat solid food again and weeks more for my stomach to accept coffee, or anything acidic. But now my normal ironclad constitution had returned and my love of caffeine had reemerged, unscathed and triumphant. Monique appeared in the doorway of the clinic, resplendent in a new teal and yellow *complet* (a wrap-around, hemmed pagne with a matching shirt and scarf), intricately embroidered around the collar with a mist of fine white thread. Her hair had been carefully woven into curly black strands, like coiled snakes. On her feet were new plastic sandals.

"What's the occasion, my friend?" I asked as I handed her a cup, then used my free hand to fend off the buzzing intruders.

"The occasion?" she said, and then noticed I was looking at her outfit. "Oh, nothing, nothing. I must go to Koutiala today, to get supplies for the clinic." She took a long swig.

Every few weeks Monique went into Koutiala to stock up on malaria pills, various injection serums, aspirin, cleaning solution, and bandages. She typically wore nicer clothes for these excursions, but never this nice. I thought of the few fancy clothes that rested in the bottom of my metal trunk: heels, a dress, even a necklace made of freshwater pearls and given to me as a college graduation gift. I had followed Peace Corps instructions and brought them along for formal embassy functions, of which I had attended exactly zero. We sipped in silence.

I looked westward where the night had retreated less than an hour earlier. Below the horizon stood my home under construction. The dark red of fresh *banco* (the mud and dung mixture used as mortar) oozed from between the light brown bricks. The sheets of corrugated tin, soon to become the roof, rested against the néré tree. My gaze wandered to the dùgùtigi's interrupted house. I, not the esteemed chief, would be the first to live in the new quartier, simply because I could afford a roof.

Progress had been faster than I'd expected. It was Ramadan, the Muslim month of fasting, during which followers could consume no water or food during daylight hours. The hardiest would not even swallow their own spit. Lucky for me, most of the men working on my future home practiced a form of Islam that was quite relaxed and demanded less rigid adherence than that practiced in other parts of the country. They could refuel throughout the day and continue to work.

An oily fly landed on my nose. Without thinking, I blew at the intruder and sprayed coffee. The bug departed only long enough to escape the spray, returning as I looked down and surveyed my wet dress. The fly dodged my swipes and landed on the exact same spot, as if connected to my right nostril by unseen elastic.

"Elise has gone to another village, in search of a husband," Monique said. "Blanche will be bringing Karamogo out here soon. At least we will be able to weigh him."

I hit my nose instead of the fly, spilled more coffee, gave up, and followed her inside.

Monique rummaged through some papers and waved Karamogo's green chart in the air. We kept it at the clinic, in the off chance Elise might show. Since we had enticed her with the prospect of a new bra six months ago, she had come to the clinic twice. Karamogo's weight had fallen just inside the red zone both times.

Soon Blanche arrived, Karamogo strapped to her back. I carefully cradled his wrinkled bum and placed him in the sling, shooing the flies away from his face, then from my own. I relayed his weight so Monique could record it. No improvement. He still teetered on the brink of severe malnutrition.

Monique spoke in Minianka to Blanche, pointing at the chart while Blanche nodded and said, "Oh." Done, she rewrapped her grandson and left.

"Elise's milk is gone and Karamogo needs to be eating more food. I make him broth when I can, but Elise and Blanche, too, need to learn to make this."

As Blanche exited, Korotun entered the doorway and greeted us.

"I am going to pound millet," she said. "I need your help, Fatumata."

She grabbed my hand and pretended to struggle and pull me. My soft hands, not toughened by the wood of any pestle, continued to be a source of light mockery.

"Sure, let's go," I said, calling her bluff. "Good-bye Monique. I'll be back in twelve hours."

She and I walked a few yards away. Then she stopped and pulled me back toward the clinic. "Thank you, thank you," she said, laughing.

"Someone is in a good mood today," I said. Monique came out onto the porch.

"Monique and Fatumata, you must both help me do my work today, for I am not well," Korotun said with a mock pout. "I have been throwing up this week and I missed my cycle last month." She bit her lip in a sassy gesture.

"Ha! There is something going on in there," Monique cried out. She looked at Korotun, then me. We slapped each other's hands.

"Korotun, it is wonderful!" I said. I took a long look at her. She was radiant.

"Koro, you must start coming to prenatal consultations," Monique said.

"I will, I will," she said. "Now I must go, but I wanted to tell you. Dramane does not want a girl, so you must both pray for me each day that I have a boy." She rubbed one hand over her belly, looked at us, turned, and left.

The remainder of the morning was routine: full of weighing babies; giving advice on vaccines, rehydration, and baby food; and treating a variety of ailments and accidents. I was glad that pregnant and nursing mothers, as well as children, were exempt from the laws of Ramadan, no matter how strict the interpretation. Monique seemed somewhat lost in thought. At noon she started putting away vials and reminded me that she must leave soon for Koutiala. She was getting a ride with Seydou, the blacksmith, on his moped. I grabbed the short-handled broom, bent over, and quickly swept the floor in wide strokes, brushing the dirt out the door with care, not wanting to spoil her outfit. Monique locked up. We sat on the corner of the porch.

"You'll be back tonight?" I asked.

"Yes, I am going to stop by my parents' house after the market, make the evening meal, and then come back." She added, "An old friend is meeting me there."

A moped engine sounded in the distance and she looked in its direction.

"Is this the old friend I have been delivering letters to?"

Now that the Peace Corps had dropped off my motorcycle, I made more trips to Koutiala for errands. Each week for the past three, Monique gave me a letter to leave with her mother. Each of these letters had the name of the mysterious recipient: Pascal.

"Yes." She had never mentioned a male friend before.

She looked down and brushed some invisible debris off her sandals. I wondered how risky it was to communicate with a man other than one's husband or male relatives, and if François knew anything about it. Another moped made its rasping presence heard. This one grew louder until it rounded the corner, and came to a stop only when the driver dragged his feet across the ground. "My ride," Monique said. We both stood up.

"Could I meet Pascal sometime?"

She sucked in her breath and nodded her head, making her coiled hair dance.

The airy hollow sound of balafons and earthy beat of drums had started at 4 AM. Monique explained that Nampossela's oldest woman, one of the Kelema clan, had died in the night. The Kelemas, at least the men, were blacksmiths, and blacksmiths had strong and ancient ties to the féticheurs, perhaps due to their work with fire and the forging of iron for tools and weapons. In most villages, the blacksmiths were the poorest of the poor, but what these families lacked in financial power they made up for in sacred connections to the supernatural world. It just so happened that the Kelemas were an enterprising lot. They invested in a blacksmith shop complete with welding torches and a generator that operated their tools. Gone were the hand bellows and crude hammers. They had done so well they owned several mopeds. In short, they had the magic and the money.

Old Woman Kelema timed her death well. If she had died during the planting or harvesting season, or even last month during Ramadan, the village would have postponed the major celebration. They all wanted to party together. Her status, and timely demise, assured a spontaneous, full day of festivities: *une fête* of music, dancing, and feasting.

Monique and I closed the clinic early; there were no patients as everyone was at the funeral. We walked past the fête in the village center on the way to Old Woman Kelema's home, located in the oldest section of the village, close to the stream and surrounded by enormous néré and baobab trees.

"We must give our *sàya fòli*—death greetings—to her family, the benedictions one gives when someone has died." Monique said as we walked. "I'll tell you some common ones: *Allah ka hiné a la*—May God have pity on the deceased. *Allah ka ye fisaya ma*—May God put him in paradise. *Allah ka dayoro sumaya*—May God cool his resting place . . ."

"Wait, stop. Let me memorize these before we arrive, so I at least have something to offer." The same blessings were used no matter what religion the person practiced. I stopped walking and repeated them to myself as Monique waited, chuckling at my earnestness.

The compound was as packed as Koutiala on market day. Men sat in clusters drinking dòlo, and kids ran about in packs. Younger women were cooking large cauldrons of rice and sauce. There was talking and laughing, but no crying. A lone white sheep, soon to be killed and eaten, was tethered to a stake near the entrance.

Under a large straw hangar, an open-air structure with a thatched roof, old women were gathered, ancient women in fact. A couple were fat and substantial, but most were frail, the sagging skin almost sloughing off to the ground. I could place the faces of about half. Many of those over seventy or eighty stuck close to their compounds. Unless they came out for a special occasion, like today, I did not see them. They sat in a rough circle while girls tended to them, bringing tea, kola nuts, dòlo, and bowls of food.

I was so besieged with greetings that it took me a couple of seconds to notice Old Woman Kelema. She was lying in the center of the circle on a mat, wrapped in pagnes, save her hands and feet. A large woman held her left hand as she talked to the corpse.

A girl came up with a chair and a wooden stool. Monique took the stool, and as soon as we were seated we were offered dòlo and food. I declined. I could not imagine eating, or drinking, and found my eyes going back to the dead limbs. Monique accepted rice and meat, swinging Basil off her back to feed him small, prechewed bits.

I had attended my first funeral just months before going into the Peace Corps. My maternal grandmother had been my favorite relative, despite her intense dislike and fears of my impending work in Africa. She was the first dead person I had ever seen. I remembered standing in front of the casket during viewing hours, wanting to make some special gesture of parting, but I couldn't lay a hand on Granny. I could look at death, in a sky blue dress, but could not touch it.

The wrapped parcel that had been Old Woman Kelema seemed so small, hardly capable of holding the remains of a life. The same large woman continued her monologue, holding the one limp hand. I couldn't make sense of the Minianka but thought I could get the gist: Where we have been, where we are, and where we are going. Where you have gone. We will follow.

Monique nudged me after eating, signaling that she was done and we could begin our death greetings. Monique gave hers and then spent a couple of minutes "introducing" me (everyone knew me, it was a formality) before I gave the one greeting I had memorized, the one that spoke to me most on this hot, dry day: *May God cool her resting place.* The old women who could hear me responded with "*Aminas*," and nodded.

"Monique, am I expected to hold the old woman's hand?"

"No. Why, do you have something you need to tell her?"

She had a slight smile.

"No, I was just wondering . . ."

"You said your benediction. To the living. That is enough. Soon it will be time to take her to the four quartiers of the village. More people will say goodbye before they run—I mean they truly run as they carry her above their heads—to the cemetery. There she will be buried, and her last serving of tŏ will be placed on the ground beside her."

Later after dinner, Monique and I followed the sound of the balafons back to the Kelema quartier. Old Woman Kelema, wrapped in an old straw mat, one arm still exposed and dangling, was held high in the air above the heads of four men. Some people approached, reached up, and swung her hand to the music. Her body dipped and swayed in ways it had not in years, I was sure. Women put their hands to their mouths and yipped and hollered.

People began to dance, and as they did the strangeness began to fade. I had never lived so close to death. Death here was not quarantined, something that only took place in slaughterhouses and hospitals, that only occasionally escaped in the form of car accidents. It was in every home, all the time. And for a person to have lived this long, in a place where life is frequently cut short, it was truly something to celebrate.

"Monique, let's dance with everyone."

"Oh, no, Fatumata, you go. Your Monique can't dance."

"What? You? Can't dance? I don't believe it," I said, grabbing her hand.

"My feet don't move like that," she said. "Even as a child, I could not dance."

"Come on," I pleaded. "It's never too late to learn how to dance."

She bent over, allowing me to pull her arm, but her feet remained planted. I looked at her and saw what amazingly looked like shyness.

"You go, Fatumata," Monique said.

I looked at the stamping and swirling feet, dropped her hand, and entered the dusty fray. I loved dancing, the faster, the better. I had trouble keeping up with the intricate rhythms, but I was quick. My feet pounded like the hooves of panicked beasts. I spun and spun, the crowd pushed back as my arms swung and my derrière pulsed. The crowd went crazy. They created a circle around me, pointing and cheering. One woman came forward, grabbed my hand and raised it high in the air. She let out a shrill cry, and others joined in. Children laughed at me, and men and women smiled and shook their heads. Panting, I rejoined Monique.

"Pati, Fatumata, you have given them a sight they will not soon forget."

"Next time, you're coming with me," I responded.

A few weeks later, the opportunity to meet Pascal presented itself. It wasn't easy for Monique to leave the village, even for an afternoon, and she could never be gone for more than a night, but today there were no women in the birthing house and she did need supplies. She hitched an early ride to Koutiala.

John was visiting again, to see me and my newly finished home. I was happy on both counts. I was glad to see John—despite my initial reservations, our romance was blossoming and he was visiting more and more often—and my new hut was quite comfortable. It had three rooms: one for storage, one for cooking and sitting (complete with a gas camping stove and a bench and chairs made by the local carpenter), and one for sleeping. There was an opening in the wall separating the living room and bedroom, the mason's mistake, but one that added a nice airy feel. The yard walls and nyegen still needed to be built. The dùgùtigi had been surprised, but acquiesced, when I insisted the workers not add the "pink powder that kills bugs" to the cement coating for my walls. Though I explained the dangers of DDT (which was available in plastic bags at almost any market), he could only sing its praise and explain that anyone he knew who could afford it, used it.

John was suitably complimentary about my homestead but was antsy to go to Koutiala and spend the night with Monique's family. He relished the thought of time in the "big city" after so many months in the bush. This would be my third time spending the night at Monique's parents' and John's first, though he had met the family on several occasions. I was also eager to finally meet Pascal.

Jeanne and Apollinaire, Monique's mother and father, lived in the northernmost section of Koutiala in a neighborhood of wide undulating dirt streets and large compounds. The tall metal gates to their compound were always open, literally and figuratively. They were also jàtigis, like Monique. They hosted a variety of students sent from outlying villages to attend school in Koutiala.

As John and I walked into the compound late that afternoon, Polici, their guard dog, ears torn and fur scarred from countless fights, came at us, teeth bared and growling. But in an instant, recognition dawned and he came bounding the rest of the way.

"Oh, Polici, Polici." John grabbed his head and got down on one knee to bond face to face. He announced that Polici had several ticks in his ears, found a scrap of cloth, and started extracting them. Polici was one of the friendliest dogs we knew. Most pets had had the friendliness beaten out of them long ago. The dogs and cats that we had met in the village seemed purely functional, owned to chase mice or protect the home, not as pets per se. Polici, like most Malian canines, was shorthaired with a tan coat. A few times I'd seen a dog with a brindled coat of brown swirled in black— uncommon, Monique had said, and used for sacrifice. Regardless of coat, most dogs were scrawny, hungry, and wary of humans. I was sure that Polici's nature meant that his owners had gentle hands.

Angele, one of Monique's younger sisters, also bounced over to greet us. Despite their ten-year age difference, Monique and Angele were identical, the same face with a wide, cheeky grin and almond eyes, and the same short, strong body. Twelve-year-old Joseph, one of Monique's round-faced and cheerful little brothers, joined us, taking a particular interest in John's hiking boots and wanting to sit on our motorcycle.

"Fatumu! Bakary! Welcome."

Monique's mother Jeanne was the only person who called me Fatumu, and I adored it. She rose slowly from her stool and held our hands. Her movements were never quick, no doubt due to having birthed twelve children over a span of twenty years, but she had the eyes of a jubilant teenager. Her smile was huge, full of glee, abandon, and crooked teeth, her face bright and smooth but for three short, dark grooves in the center of her forehead.

I sat down on a wooden stool in the shade next to Jeanne. Once, I had asked her about her facial scars, and she told me that she made these marks on a whim as a young girl, cutting identity into her face just as her ancestors had done. She had said that a long time ago, everyone in the village had markings like these, so that no matter where a person went, he knew his people. In the time of slavery, the markings helped people find each other. The three lines on her forehead showed that she came from the region of Karangasso. She had then explained that if I wished to be a true Minianka, I would have to do the same. I then called for a knife, which sent everyone into hysterics.

Now, I called for a knife to help peel potatoes. Monique emerged from the smoke-filled doorway of the cooking hut, tripping over a gourd bowl of water in the process, startling the half-asleep Basil on her back. She dropped her face for a second in a mock gesture of embarrassment. She worked as hard here as she did in Nampossela, preparing meals and cleaning, but her heart was obviously lighter. Monique had toiled since she was young, as four brothers were born after her and not one sister to help with the chores. It had meant that she had to leave school in the sixth grade to attend to domestic duties, while her brothers continued. Monique had said, laughing, that her brothers had been forced to carry water, peel millet, and sweep because there was no one else to do the work. That they would make good husbands because of this. I thought she was right, but wondered how long she would have continued in school if she'd had less work.

"You have come, you have come," Monique announced, looking at John. "Bakary, you are here. *C'est bon.* The lettuce is bought, Bakary is here, the big party can begin!" She brought a knife and another bowl and placed them beside me. But before I could touch the utensil, Monique stilled my hand and whispered in my ear.

"Fatumata, come. I have something for you."

She pulled me into a hut and plopped Basil on a mat. The concrete floor looked recently mopped, and the dark corners were free of dust.

"Here is what Apollinaire made for you."

Monique's father was a tailor, and highly adept with a foot-powered sewing machine. I unfolded the wrap-around skirt, a pagne in a bold purple-and-blue leaf pattern and a matching shirt with puffy sleeves, silver-dollar-size buttons, and a wide flower petal collar. I ran my fingers across the smooth material, realizing that it had been carefully pressed with an iron heated over hot coals.

"Monique, this is beautiful."

"Look at the corners, Fatumata."

I unfolded the corners of the skirt and unraveled long thin pieces of fabric.

"When young girls are first learning how to wear a pagne, sometimes we sew straps onto the corners so the pagne can be tied and doesn't fall down if they don't wrap it right. He thought you might need them."

"Oh, Monique, you didn't tell your father, did you?"

I had come perilously close to showing the village my underwear several times, most recently a couple of weeks ago. My pagne had loosened and begun a slow plummet while I was trying to balance a bucket of pump water on my head. I stopped walking, and the pagne stopped sliding. Monique simply stared. Suddenly, the pagne dropped. With a shriek I caught it just in time, but at the expense of gallons of water spilling everywhere. Monique had to put down her own bucket for laughing so hard. We spent that evening going over the fine details of pagne wrapping—again—a technique that I could not master even after ten months in Mali. Now I could finally wear one without fear.

"Don't worry. No one can see the straps," she said.

I went into an adjoining room to put on my blouse and "training" pagne. I walked back out and as a test, spread my legs wide and jumped up and down. I pretended to hold something on my head and skipped across the room, raising my knees to aerobic heights. Everything held. Basil stared from the mat and howled for Monique to save him.

"Ah, you are becoming a true Mali *muso*—woman," Monique said, letting Basil hide between her legs. She took off her working shirt, under which she had on her black bra, and looked at two other shirts, one white and one black, laid out on the mat near Basil. She rubbed scented lotion onto her arms and neck as she contemplated her wardrobe.

"Which one?"

"That one," I said, choosing the gaudier of the two, a wide-necked white shirt with shiny plastic daisies strung along the collar. Monique pulled it on and adjusted it to expose one bra strap.

"And now these." She carefully held up a necklace of fake gold beads strung on a pink plastic string and turned around for me to fasten it.

"Wait a minute," I said, and unzipped the side pocket of my backpack on the floor. I knew she had a weakness for sequins, glitter, and embellishments. I had remembered the pearl necklace.

"Here, you can wear this tonight."

"Oh, Fatumata! What are these?"

"I don't know the word in French. They are made by . . . by . . ." I couldn't remember the French word for oyster either, "by animals that live in water. They take sand and turn it into these."

"These are made from sand? What a good idea," she said as she moved the three entwined strands of pearls in her hand and watched them catch the light, their iridescence changing with each subtle movement of her fingers. "Ah, ah, they are so pretty. You are sure you want to let me wear this?"

"Yes," I said, fastening the gold clasp behind her neck. "It's perfect for this most special of nights."

She then wrapped a crisp black scarf around her head, tying it so the ends fanned out in back like a peacock's tail, strapped the now calm Basil on with a clean, white pagne, and smiled.

"Voilà. I am ready for our trip to the movies."

"The movies? Wow, Bakary will love it."

I had not been to the popular outdoor movie theatre in Koutiala, but I had heard they showed mostly pirated American action thrillers and Hong Kong kung-fu flicks.

I walked back outside in confident, long strides. Angele was preparing our eating area with some final flicks of a broom. The stiff straws left long scratches in the dirt. A hen the color of fresh corn followed and pecked at the ground, while her three chicks scurried about, vaguely imitating her. John sat on stool while Geneviève, Monique's daughter, leaned next to him, chewing on a potato peel, big belly resting on her thighs.

"Monique, you look incredible! But couldn't you have done something with Fatumata?" John asked.

"Hey!" Monique lunged at him and pretended to slap his face, complete with sound effects. Gené giggled heartily.

"At least I am wearing a pagne that won't fall down," I said and began to strut around.

"That's too bad," John said, and Monique pointed a warning finger at him.

"Good evening," said a deep voice from the entrance to the compound.

I stopped my strutting. Apollinaire walked smartly across the yard with a tall man in uniform. Apollinaire's erect stature, angular face, and tiny eyes always looked so harsh, but his light step and outstretched arms radiated warmth and friendliness. I had never seen the other fellow. He wore a crisp khaki uniform with a green beret, both of which displayed the red, yellow, and green shield of the Republic of Mali.

Monique's eyes widened. She bit her bottom lip. "Good evening," she breathed.

That told me everything.

"Fatumata and Bakary, it has been too long," Apollinaire said, and smiled when he saw my outfit. "Fatumata, I hope you like your clothes."

"Yes, thanks," I said, "they're really beautiful."

"Fatumata and Bakary, my name is Pascal. Pascal Konaté. Pleased to meet you."

He stepped toward us, bowed slightly as he took John's outstretched hand in his, and repeated the gesture with me. With his large, darting eyes, long nose, and softly drooping mouth, he looked like a tamed raptor.

"Get them seats," Monique instructed her younger sisters. Little Natalie, the youngest, and at five years old, barely Gené's senior, came forward bearing a large wooden stool on her head that she flipped over on the ground.

As Pascal sat down, seven-year-old Urbain, yet another of Monique's brothers, began to sneak up behind him. Pascal looked over his shoulder then threw his hands behind his back and grabbed the child around the waist.

"I've got you, Urbain!"

Urbain squealed in delight.

"Pascal is in the army," Monique said, "and he works at the prison in town."

"Yes. I am a guard," he said.

"A prison in Koutiala, I had no idea. What do people . . ." John said. I knew he was searching for the right French words. "What do people do to end up in prison here?"

"A few of our prisoners have killed someone, but most are thieves. Most are caught here, in Koutiala. In the bush, village justice is usually enough. The chief and his counsel decide what happens. They may give the person a warning, or they make him give back what he took and perform a service to the wronged family. Sometimes the person just loses face and other times he is beaten and driven from the community."

Now there's a deterrent, I thought. Community is everything here.

"What do you do in the army?" John asked. I looked at the bands and buttons that decorated his khaki lapel, indicators of his military status.

"I am infantry, on reserve."

"So, you work for General Traoré?" John asked.

"Yes." Pascal laughed.

Since 1968, Mali had been under the one-man rule of Moussa Traoré. The aging general's portrait hung everywhere, in banks, homes, and stores, as if his sheer paper presence and harsh stare were enforcing his will.

"What do you think of the recent protests in Bamako?"

"The protests?" Pascal thought this over for a moment. Urbain took advantage of the pause and came in for another attack. Pascal caught his little prisoner by the arm, pulled him into his lap, and then continued. "Students are talking democracy again. People are upset. But General Traoré is not worried. He has been in power for over twenty years. The students tried this in 1981 and they did not succeed. They will not succeed now."

Not succeed? Not only did they not succeed in 1981, but also from what I knew of Malian history, the demonstrators had been swiftly and brutally crushed. Mali had yet to taste anything close to free speech or democracy. But I didn't want to get into a political debate with Monique's special friend.

"So, do you like being a prison guard?" I asked.

"*Oui.* I joined the army, I've been here and there, and this is where I am now. It is not easy being an honest guard. People do everything so we will release them. The things I get offered each day! Money, clothes, cassettes of music. Truthfully, it is not very exciting, but it is good to be back home."

I didn't want to ask whether he actually allowed prisoners to buy their freedom. I wanted to like him. While we awaited dinner, Pascal talked and joked, went into the house briefly with Apollinaire, went to the nyegen, and into the cooking hut where Monique and Angele were, seemingly comfortable with every corner.

The four of us ate out of the same bowl, Monique and Pascal next to each other, knees touching, sharing their food and space in a way I was sure Monique and François never had. When dinner was through, we walked to the show. The theater had high mud walls and huddles of people outside the door. We paid the equivalent of thirty cents each to enter total chaos.

The spacious compound was filled with people greeting one another, jostling for seats. The air was full of the smells of hot food and the shouts of scampering children. A huge rectangle of plywood hung on one wall and an old 16-mm projector, powered by a gas generator, sat on a spindly table behind uneven rows of weathered benches and flimsy chairs. As foreigners and the hosts of foreigners, we were given chairs in the front row. Monique and I sat in the middle, Pascal and John flanking us.

Tonight's movie, *Terminator*, was perfectly confusing. Deep-voiced Arnold Schwarzenegger spoke falsetto French, though it was hard to hear anything over the generator. The six reels were shown out of order; characters died then reappeared, and the final scene took place around reel two. No one seemed to care. They cheered at the fights and gasped at the suspense.

Monique and Pascal weren't watching the movie at all. They sank down in their chairs, their heads leaning together, engaged in conversation, while Basil slept in Monique's arms. I heard Pascal's voice turn creamy and deep and saw her touch his arm. I caught John's eye and pointed to Monique and Pascal. Not wanting to be left out of any action, he grabbed my hand and held it.

On the way out of the theater, Pascal asked if all Hollywood movies were this strange. As we explained the intended storyline we drew quite a crowd. Malians were always eager to learn more about the United States. Tonight they wanted to know how we survived in such a violent country. As we entered the family's compound, Pascal stopped just outside the doorway and said, "Thank you for the evening. I hope to see you another time. You must come out to my prison one day and have a tour."

"I'd like that," John replied. I wasn't so sure.

"I am coming soon," Monique said to us, moving next to Pascal. "Good night."

Yawning, John took my hand. We walked across the deserted yard and crept into the room where we were staying. Two straw mats with two straw pillows were laid out.

"What do you think about all this?" I whispered, not wanting to wake the rest of the family. They were sleeping together in the two neighboring rooms, as they'd vacated the largest one for us.

"They are quite an item, I'd say."

"Yes, and she's ecstatic!" I said. "*I* am happy just seeing her like this."

"Do you think François knows?"

"Doubtful. He stays in the village, pretty much."

Despite my good mood, John's mention of François sent a shiver through me that I could not ignore. It did not seem uncommon for married men to have girlfriends, but the girlfriends were always young and single. What was the penalty for infidelity with another married person? Village justice? I was not concerned about Pascal for I figured men always got off the hook, but what about a married woman with a boyfriend?

John yawned again, rolled onto his side and fell asleep. I tried to be productive and picked up my copy of the village health care manual I had been reading, *Where There Is No Doctor*. I looked at it by flashlight, but succeeded only in wasting my precious batteries as I thought about Monique and Pascal. I supported her seeing him because her marriage had nothing to do with love. And she wasn't spending money on Pascal, buying him fancy watches or numerous Castel beers, thereby diverting precious resources from the family. But what of François and his girlfriends? I doubted I would support him no matter how well behaved he was about it. After an hour or so of pondering, I heard soft footsteps outside the curtain that covered our doorway. I pushed it aside and peeked out. Monique was sitting down, moving a sleepy Basil off her back and onto the straw mat. Despite my insistence she could sleep in our room, she was bunking in the foyer.

"Ahh, Fatumata, I thought I saw light in your room. It is late for you."

Basil sat up for a moment, giving me a brief heavy lidded stare and scowl before lying back down. I came out and settled alongside her, letting the moonlight flood through the open door and bathe us in quivering blue.

"You seem to be very happy with Pascal."

"He is a friend from childhood, we have been best friends since we were kids."

"And you couldn't marry because your marriage was already arranged . . ."

"Yes, mine was arranged, as was his," she said and turned her face toward me, as if reading my mind. The pearl necklace glistened. "What's done is done. Here, the children belong to their father. If I leave le gars, I must leave them. I cannot do that. So voilà, you see my situation. Fatumata, if it were not for you and Bakary, Pascal and I would not have had permission to pass this evening together."

Her eyes pierced the dark, a deep, vivid brown, gauging my reaction. "With you here, it's okay."

She needn't have searched for my blessing. She had it.

Over the following weeks we fell into the routine of seeing Pascal whenever possible. Though John was back in his village, it seemed fine for Monique and me to go out together with Pascal when we were in Koutiala. I enjoyed his laid-back demeanor and relished the late-night chats with Monique after everyone else was asleep. Of course, Monique always woke early the next morning feeling refreshed and alive. Never a night owl, I would sleep in, not stirring until a lazy 8 AM. Then I would squint at a world that was already in full swing: pans clattering, kids yelling, and donkeys braying.

"Almost time to leave for church," Monique said, shaking me awake one Sunday morning.

Monique loved going to the Catholic church in Koutiala. It was a much grander place than the one in Nampossela. The mile and a half walk there wound through the wide, red-dirt streets. Monique and I ambled along while Basil wiggled uncomfortably on her back. We'd had a light rain in the night, and the morning was filled with the earth's moist, pungent breath. Vendors selling breakfasts of coffee, bananas, and egg-and-bread sandwiches lined the road, and my stomach growled, despite my breakfast of millet porridge.

Farther along the roadside, four children gathered around the trunk of a large mango tree while two others ascended its branches. In fact, the entire row of mango trees lining the road was alive with children. Plump and sweet, the large oval fruits dangled like Christmas decorations, orange and gold treats beckoning bird and beast alike.

"Look at the child in that tree over there, picking those unripe mangoes," Monique said. "His stomach hopes so much that it will be ripe and soft that his eyes refuse to see it is green and hard. Oh, will he have konoboli tonight."

She tilted her wide face up to the sky, arms holding her belly in mock pain. She could laugh at the sour stomach that comes from impatience, altogether different from the diarrhea that kills.

"How can you blame him?" I said. "The only ripe ones left are way up on the highest limbs of the tree. The poor kid would kill himself trying to climb that far up."

Monique stopped in her tracks and cocked her head at me.

"Ah, Fatumata, so you don't think anyone can get those ripe ones up there?"

I sensed a challenge.

"Oh, no, there is no way I am going up there," I said, laughing. "And if you start climbing up there, my friend, your pagne will certainly fall off and the sun will shine where it should not."

"I can get those mangoes, dear Fatumata. And without losing my pagne!"

"I dare you."

Monique walked to the roadside, searching the ground. She picked up a few rocks, tested their weight, and tossed them back. After a minute she found a suitable projectile, a stone the size of her fist, and walked back toward the tree. The girls and boys tumbled out of the branches and stood at a respectful distance.

"Now you watch the great lady Monique in action," she said.

Just to be safe, she rewrapped and retucked her pagne. Squinting up at the tree's top, she planted her thonged feet on solid ground, drew back her right arm, and hurled the stone. It arced through the air with formidable speed, missing everything. Not a branch was touched. Monique stared in disbelief.

"Well, lady, you have proven your strength, but not your aim."

She raised an eyebrow in my direction and went straight to finding another stone. The group of children stepped farther back from the tree, murmuring among themselves. Armed with a second stone, Monique once again faced the tree. This had become a personal battle between flora and female. She stared at the branch a long time, then took aim and fired.

The thud of victory was sweet, and the ripe mangoes came tumbling down through the leaves.

"Yuh! Yuh!" Monique yelled as she hopped over to retrieve them. The crowd of children yelled with her. She waltzed back, did a mock curtsy, and presented one to me as if I were a queen and she the commissioned hunter returning with the kill. I accepted graciously. She took a mango for herself and gave the rest to the giggling kids. We ripped open the thin skins with our teeth and fingers and bit into the fleshy meat.

"This mango is so sweet," I said, jutting my chin out as the juice dribbled off of it and onto the sand. "Thank you, my dear Monique."

"It is the mango rains that we must thank."

"Mango rains?"

"The small rains that come, in February and March. They come when the earth is dry and the heavy rains still far away to make the mangoes sweet," Monique said, wiping the delicious stickiness off her face. "You do not remember?"

Yes, I did, I nodded. The brief rains that fell when I least expected them.

We discarded the pits and turned onto the main road—called a "highway" simply because it was paved—that traveled northeast, passing the market town of San and bumping into the border of Burkina Faso. It was abuzz with fast-moving trucks and whirring mopeds. Just beyond the busy road was a large yellowed concrete building surrounded by verandas. A stained wall contained the vast complex. I looked for a cross.

"Is that it?" I asked Monique, as we carefully crossed the highway.

"No, no. The church is farther up the road. This building is the Koutiala hospital and maternity ward. It is where I gave birth to my children, where I did my training."

I thought about the birthing house in Nampossela. This building was so much bigger, a modern, Western-style edifice in comparison. But there was nothing soft or welcoming about it, nothing to make me feel that birth was somehow safer here. It seemed a barren place, not at all one in which life was renewed.

When we finally arrived at the church, there was no mistaking it. The huge A-frame structure had a towering, rusted metal cross on its peak. As we got closer, greetings rang out from all directions. Monique was quickly surrounded. She laughed, slapped hands, and asked questions of her old friends and neighbors. She positively glowed. Someone yelled from within the church, a signal that the service was about to begin.

The sanctuary was spacious and rugged, free of the stained glass, deep red carpets, cushioned pews, and religious paintings I associated with churchgoing. The whitewashed walls were reddened with dust, and the floor was lined with row upon row of wooden benches filled with parishioners. Men sat in one section, women and children in another. I looked for Jeanne, who had come earlier with Monique's younger siblings and Gené, but could not find them in the sea of headscarves. We sat down. The pulpit was a simple white stand. Behind it, an enormous window was held in place by a crisscrossed metal frame, creating the illusion of hundreds of connected crucifixes.

I was beat from the night before, and didn't follow all the Bambara. Although the rhythm of the service—short Bible verses, intermittent songs, and a long sermon—was familiar, the hymns sung to the balafon, the unbridled enthusiasm of the congregation, and the segregation by sex were foreign to me. It appeared that Catholicism had picked up a distinctive Malian flavor.

Monique was absorbed in the ceremony, lost in it. Eyes closed, she prayed, she sang. I stayed seated when Monique rose to take communion. She did not just partake, she relished the blood and flesh; there was nothing subtle or reserved about it. My ancestors had been Christians for hundreds of years, but Christianity was still fresh for her and her family.

After the service we walked outside into the churchyard. Joseph, Monique's brother, clad in a white robe, was among the acolytes gathered there. Monique had said that she was sure he would become a priest one day. We greeted several Malian priests and one or two aging *Pères Blancs*, "White Fathers," the French missionary priests who had founded the congregation. Then we made our way to Angele who was leaning against one of the huge trees that lined the churchyard, talking with a group of teenage girls. Gené was with her and waved to us.

"How long has your family been Catholic?" I asked Monique.

"My grandfather, the father of Apollinaire, converted. It was a long time ago, just after the first Malian in Koutiala became Christian, in nineteen thirty-six."

"Thirty-six?"

"Yes, I can still remember the date from church school."

"The service here was similar to those in my town," I said, "but the atmosphere, the music, the language, of course, were all very different."

"You attend church in your village, in the United States?"

"Yes, I used to go, with my family. It was a Protestant church, called Presbyterian."

"Presbyterian? I don't think we have those here."

"Maybe not. I never actually joined it. I went because my family went and I had friends there, but I was never sure what I believed in."

"Not to worry, Fatumata," she said. "It is all the same if you pray to one God or another, because it is the same God. All religions are the same. But for me, it is the Christians who give more. It is the Christians who believe in helping the poor. Why else would our White Fathers and Sisters have come all the way from your lands to Mali, eh?"

"That, I don't know," I said. "The missionaries here certainly are devoted to what they're doing, but sometimes they seem more concerned with saving people after death than helping them in this life."

Missionaries were not all the same. The Catholic missionaries, most of them from France, allowed for some mixing in of traditional beliefs, such as letting people wear protective amulets, even in church. One could sacrifice a chicken every now and again, and not be excommunicated. On the other hand, the Protestant missionaries, most of them from the United States, represented a stricter Christianity. One was either saved or not, born-again or not. No shades of acceptance.

Monique and I sat next to Gené under the dappled shadow of a huge old néré tree. Angele and her friends had run off, and Gené looked after them sadly, but became distracted by a piece of rubber tire lying on the ground, which she began stuffing into an empty powdered milk can. Behind her was a wide trail that wound through a field and disappeared over a knoll. Dotting the distant hillsides behind it were mounds and mounds of heaved earth.

"Is that a graveyard?" I asked.

"Yes, for Catholics." There were no stone markers, no iron gates, just piles of dirt like the burial ground in Nampossela; only this was so much bigger.

Monique swept her hand back and forth across the horizon in firm strokes. "This is where my family is buried. Grandparents, aunts, uncles, my two brothers, and my first son."

"You had a child before Gené?" Gené looked up at the mention of her name.

"Yes, his name was Louis, named for François' father, his *togoma*. He was two years old when he died. He was very sick and had awful diarrhea. It was before my training, so I did not know what to do. I was way out in Nampossela."

"I'm so sorry."

Little Louis. A lost child. I wondered how many children she had saved since then.

One morning, as I made my way toward the Dembele family compound to get Monique, I heard the sputtering of an approaching moped. François rounded the corner and swung down the narrow path toward me. Frightened by his speed and erratic steering, I flattened myself against the wall as he blew past in a cloud of blue smoke.

"Asshole," I muttered in English, and entered the family compound.

Monique came from inside one of the huts. She had her medical bag packed, and Basil tightly secured on her back.

"Fatumata, I am on my way out." She closed the hut door behind her.

"Aren't we going to do baby food demonstrations?"

"You will have to do them. I have to get out to a hamlet of the Koné family to attend a woman in labor. And I must find a ride," she said, bustling ahead. "Le gars has taken the moped again. Did you not see him?"

"Yes, I saw him. Can't the village tell François to let you have it?" I huffed as I tried to keep pace with her. For a short woman, she certainly had a large stride. "The village bought it for your work, right?"

"No, Fatumata, I must ask him if I want to use it. Can't you see how proud he is to be seen on it? It is a great machine for a great man. It has become more important than his radio, or his jean clothes."

"Could you buy another one?" I asked.

"Ah, it is complicated. The old one, Louis, he does not give me enough money to save a thing."

"Why does Louis give you money? I thought you had a salary."

"Louis collects my salary, 11,500 CFA each month, from Adama."

"You don't pick up your own salary?"

"No, no, no."

I calculated the amount: twenty-three dollars, less than a dollar per day. A donkey cart driver made more than Monique did. But donkey cart drivers were men. Then to receive only a fraction of this pay... My mind swam with questions and protests, all of which were drowned out as a mufflerless moped roared into view. Strapped to its miniscule rack was a large white goat—too crowded for Monique to hitch a ride on. Man and machine suddenly swerved in a patch of sand when the driver waved to us, but quickly righted. The frantic bleats of the hapless beast were silenced against the engine's racket. Monique stopped as we entered the main artery leading out of town toward the clinic and toward Koutiala. Basil, still asleep, turned his head but kept his eyes closed. The cheek that had been resting against his mother's back was flat.

I fiddled with my dress, looking at the ground and trying to keep myself from getting worked up. "Has it been this way since the beginning?"

"Yes."

"But Louis didn't work for the money, Monique."

A sigh escaped her.

"The old one did not want me to take this job in the first place. The dùgùtigi had to convince him that it was a good thing for the family. The old one thinks the job just takes me away from housework."

"But you still do all the work in the family anyway! You just work longer hours than anyone else." I took my eyes off the dirt and faced her.

She met my gaze and clicked the back of her throat.

"How does the old one know what to spend the money on, what the family needs?"

Monique braced her hands on her hips.

"He does not. That isn't something for him to worry about. He gives me what he wants to give me, and I assure you, Fatumata, it is very little."

I could picture Louis, sharing kola nuts and reconstituted wine with the old men as they passed their twilight years beneath the shade of a straw hangar.

"How would it work if a man was earning the money? How much would he give his wife?" I asked.

"Normally it would be divided in half."

"But this is not what happens for you."

"Not at all," she said. "I am so sick of this family! Some days I just want to leave and never come back. Do you know what François told me this morning, when we fought over the moped? He said that it is the old one who refuses to let him divorce me. Ha!" She threw her arm into the air. "Really this is not true. It is he himself who doesn't wish it. Without me, he would not find his radio, his jeans, and the moped. Without me, he would find nothing."

I rubbed the center of my forehead with my fingers. My opinion of Louis was muddied. I felt that taking Monique's salary was wrong, yet I did not feel that he was a bad man. The truth was that almost any Malian father-in-law, as patriarch, would do the same. Resources flowed upward in families here, with belongings and money gathering at the top. But François . . . I felt he was being selfish and unfair, even by village standards.

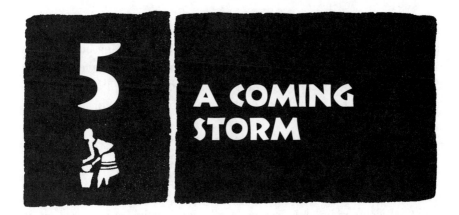

5 A COMING STORM

THE RAINS HAD COME. The clack and lurch of donkey carts laden with people and basins of food bound for the fields became constant. Paths were congested. Everyone had a *dàba* (stubby-handled hoe) across his or her shoulders, the sharp wide blade facing back, the handle forward across the chest. Time to sow by hand the precious seeds saved from last year's harvest. Every year it was a bit of a gamble, deciding when to sow the seeds. Plant too late and growing time would be lost. Too early, before the earth receives sufficient rainfall, and the shoots would die. Many villagers had not the stock to reseed, and no one could afford to make the same mistake twice. I had learned that Malians could be a laid-back folk, except about rain. As Monique said, "Rain means that people live."

Everyone was exhausted at night from the day's labor. Gone were the sounds of the balafon and the radio. Even the belotte players ceased their nightly game. In the midst of this toil and quiet came *Tabasci* or *Eid al-Adha* in Arabic, "Festival of the Sacrifice." This Muslim holiday (also fondly known in Mali as *La Fête des Moutons* or "Festival of the Sheep") takes place every year, seventy days after the end of Ramadan, to celebrate the Prophet Abraham's willingness to sacrifice his only son Ishmael at God's command. It also celebrates the return of the faithful from the Hajj, the annual pilgrimage to Mecca, which few Malians I knew made, but was revered nonetheless. Sheep, which villagers had been fattening up for months, were sliced, skinned, gutted, chopped, and sautéed all in one day. Bowl upon bowl of rice and sauce laden with fresh mouton, a feast five times more than what any family could consume, was delivered to all family compounds.

Monique and Elise didn't have to cook a meal for days. Children, dressed in their finest attire, came in and out of the compound giving benedictions and blessings. In turn, we invited them to eat and gave them a few coins or *Sogosogo bonbons*, a local cough drop that served as candy. It felt like abundance, food and health and blessings, in a time of not enough.

The birthing house was humid, stifling hot, and crowded. In the darkened front hall, women lined the cracked walls, some sitting, some standing, all with bulging bellies, all with toddlers hugging their legs, all waiting to be seen for prenatal consultations by Monique.

I murmured greetings as I made my way toward the examination room. So many women here, despite the fact that it was the rainy season, the season of constant, never-ending toil. I looked down, carefully stepping over legs, baskets, and children, and almost collided with Korotun.

"I ni sogoma, Fatumata," she said, and then scolded, "you missed my prenatal visit."

"Sorry, I had no idea there would be so many women this early." I was also tired. Bintou, a short, light-skinned woman, had gone into labor late in the evening. I had stayed with Monique in Bintou's airless hut, in the middle of a compound teeming with children, as she slowly labored on a straw mat spread out on the smooth dirt floor. Though Bintou's cervix had dilated early in the evening, she was not able to push; the contractions came and went, but she could not put force behind them. After midnight Monique insisted I get some rest, and off I went, leaving her and Bintou alone in the darkened womb of mud.

"Of course we are here early, we must get to our fields, after all. Anyway, Monique says everything is fine. But you had better not be late when it is time for me to give birth."

She pointed her finger at me for emphasis.

"I won't, Korotun, I won't."

I entered the last room on the left. Monique was leaning over a large upright metal scale, fiddling with the silver weights on the twin bars while a very pregnant woman stood motionless. Monique's temples, and Basil's sleeping head flat against her back, were beaded in moisture.

"Good, good," Monique said, giving the smaller weight a final tap. "You are gaining."

She wiped her forehead with her arm and asked the woman to lie down, then lifted the woman's shirt. The swollen belly was taut, but wrinkled and scarred; she had given birth before, many times. Using her hands as guides, Monique felt and pushed, measuring from the pubic bone to the top of the body inside.

"And the baby is growing too."

Her fingers searched through shifting skin to determine the baby's position. Strapping on a fetascope, a funny instrument that looked more musical than medical with a large cone protruding from its forehead band, she leaned over and pressed the cone down in several places until she found the baby's heartbeat.

"Your baby's head is down, which is good. He sounds strong," She took her ledger and pen off the windowsill and began to write.

Finally Monique looked at me. Her eyes were puffy and lined, evidence of a long night.

"Fatumata, hello. The blood pressure cuff is over there, if you want to help the next mother."

I grabbed the cuff and called to the next woman, who was standing just outside the doorway. She was a young woman from the Dembele quartier. I had seen her a number of times, pounding millet under the hangar. I wrapped the blood pressure cuff around her arm and began pumping it up.

"All done, Salimata," Monique said to the woman still lying down on the bed, "but watch the salt. Your blood pressure is higher than before. Drink lots of clean water. Now that you are in your last month of pregnancy, I want you to come in each week. Any questions?"

Salimata shook her head.

I listened to the rhythmic thumping of blood, watched the needle bounce, then let the air in the cuff hiss out.

"One-fifteen over seventy-five," I announced as I unwrapped the cuff, and then took the woman's pulse. "Seventy-two."

"Good." Monique recorded the numbers. Salimata sat up on the bed while the young Dembele woman got up on the scale.

"I feel a storm coming," Monique said and glanced up at the ripped edge of the roof and the holes. No repairs had been made in years. One bad tempest could peel off the entire top of the building.

Out the slatted window the sky was a brilliant blue, but a gray band hugged the western horizon. It was my first full rainy season here, but I, too, was learning to feel the coming rain. The air was pregnant with it. The heat and water, too heavy for the sky to hold, would soon be dropped.

There were at least twenty more women to see.

Salimata stood and rearranged her pagne. Monique motioned for the young woman to lie down, and then came over to the window.

"The mother, Bintou, died last night, Fatumata," she whispered. "After giving birth."

"Oh, Monique. I'm so sorry." I leaned back against the wall with a thud.

"She finally pushed her baby out, but afterwards the bleeding would not stop. I tried everything, everything . . ."

Monique rubbed her eyes, retied sleeping Basil, and returned to her work.

I stared out the slatted window. I had yet to hear of Monique losing a mother, though statistically I knew women in Mali died in labor every day, especially teen mothers whose bodies weren't ready yet for the toll of childbirth, and many-times-over mothers, like Bintou, whose bodies were worn out from it. I knew what Monique must have done last night. If putting the baby to Bintou's breast hadn't stopped the flow of blood after birth, she would have given her a shot of Pitocin, a drug that made the uterus contract and was Monique's only recourse in the event of hemorrhage. It obviously hadn't been enough.

In the handful of births I had attended, all the women and their babies had been fine, meaning that they lived, not that they were free of complications. During the pushing, some women tore horribly and then had to get stitched up. Many lost a lot of blood and many sustained a variety of infections after birth. Having spent all of my post-puberty years actively avoiding pregnancy and therefore childbirth, I was reading an old copy of *Our Bodies, Ourselves* by the Boston Women's Health Collective to educate myself. Much of the information Monique had already taught me: a woman must eat iron-rich foods and have regular prenatal check-ups; she must be in a comfortable position for the birth, be surrounded by supportive caregivers, be hydrated, and relax between contractions.

From what I was reading, it seemed that this age-old wisdom had been forgotten in hospitals in the U.S., where technology and interventions were the norm. I was astounded at the rate of Cesarean sections (around one quarter of all births) in such a healthy, rich country (could they all really be necessary?), and at the control that the medical establishment had assumed over the birthing process. In contrast, birth in Nampossela was a family and community event and lacked almost all modern medical interventions. Monique had simple tools, clean hands, and a sharp mind. But if a woman needed an IV, or a Cesarean section, or a fetal monitor, it was not an option. If Monique had had access to more emergency medical care, could she have saved Bintou? I didn't know. But I hoped that giving birth didn't have to happen at one extreme or the other—that a happy medium existed between the two.

In Mali, the rainy season was the hardest time to be pregnant and give birth, and not just because women like Bintou were forced to labor in their small, stuffy huts. Fieldwork was physically exhausting and infectious diseases abundant. Perhaps Bintou had been malnourished, fighting malaria or some other infection. Perhaps her uterus could no longer contract after bearing six children. Perhaps her husband or her heavy workload did not allow her to rest during her pregnancy or did not allow her to attend prenatal consultations, where she could have learned about taking care of herself. At least if we repair this maternity ward, I thought to myself, women can stay here before their births, and after to rest. A well-rested mother had less post-partum bleeding; she was stronger and healed faster.

I turned back from the window. Monique had measured the young woman's taut, smooth belly, felt for the baby's position, and was strapping on the fetascope.

I looked at the flawless, bright skin of the soon-to-be mother on the bed and thought of the lined, wizened leather of Salimata's stomach. Salimata stood in the doorway talking to the other women. Undoubtedly they knew about Bintou's death. Were they talking about it? About how death could just as easily visit them? Did they understand what they could do to stack the odds in their favor? Or was it simply the will of God?

"Fatumata," a small voice said from behind me. I turned to see Oumou, the well digger's wife, peeking through the doorway, over the heads of children.

She stepped a little closer, nervously smiling through her right hand, which partially covered her mouth. She had huge eyes, a long oval chin, and a flattened nose. I never stood too close to her, partly because of her shyness, partly due to the fear that she would topple over on me. Oumou had tall legs for a short woman, tall legs that bent forward so that her torso hovered backwards over and behind her rear. A hefty baby on her back made the list more alarming. She looked as if she might fall on her back at any moment.

"Come on in," Monique said.

Oumou shuffled forward, two little children hiding between her legs, and stood quietly next to me. She patted her belly under the swirls of white and green pagne. "I am here for . . ."

"You're pregnant?"

"Uh-hum," she said with her hand back over her mouth.

I looked at her from a couple of angles. I couldn't tell the difference between early pregnancy and its first swell of promise, and the leftover droopy bulge from previous children. Monique finished with the young woman and penned Oumou's name on what was now the last line in the ledger. The spaces to the right of her name were empty: a clean, hopeful slate.

Out of the corner of my eye I caught sight of Oumou falling backwards. I spun around with arms outstretched, but she was only sitting down. I let out a breath, my arms falling to my sides. Then I wrapped the blood pressure cuff around her bicep. Her children stayed at her legs. Monique called in another woman; I maneuvered to make room. Sweat fell off my brow, splattering the blood pressure gauge. Between the humidity and the warmth of the bodies, the unventilated building had to be 110 degrees.

After another hour of weighing and measuring, assessing nutrition, and extracting promises of rest and no heavy lifting, the crowd of women noticeably lessened, but not just because of us. They were leaving before the storm. A breeze found its way inside and fluttered the collar of my dress. Monique sighed. I stepped out into the emptying corridor and walked toward the open door, drawn by the hint of coolness. Dark clouds raced in the sky.

Outside, women were walking fast as they carried their laundry, fetched water, or balanced firewood on their heads. Men sped by on bicycles. Drivers hollered at their donkeys to move the carts faster (donkeys being donkeys, this had little effect). A group of girls approached, coming from the fields, singing, and dancing, energized by the electric feel of the air. Dust swirled by in eddies, wrapping around their legs before dissolving and mixing together again downwind.

"Fatumata," Oumou called as she walked out of the hallway and into the doorway.

"You're still here? I thought you had left."

"I was waiting for you to finish your work." Her eyes filled with water. "Yesterday, I lost Soloman."

"Oh, Oumou, another child died?" She had buried Gwewa only months ago.

"I cannot have more children, Fatumata, please." Her hand stilled her mouth but could not hide her desperation.

Monique quietly joined us; it was obvious that she had already heard the news.

"I lose them. I had nine. Now I am left with five and this one," Oumou pointed to her belly. "Too many have died, and yet my husband, Daouda, he wants to have more. I can't have more, Fatumata."

I searched for words in Bambara, "There are plastic things that Daouda can put on himself, and pills you can take."

"I do not have money."

"We'll see, Oumou," Monique said. "There may be something we can do, where you don't need to have money."

I wondered how much Monique knew about modern contraception.

"Hmm," Oumou said and nodded. "Daouda cannot know."

With that, she left. We watched her walk into the village, along the now deserted path, silent children in tow. They buried their faces in her tattered dress to escape the wind. Korotun wanted children, Oumou didn't. Both wanted control over situations where they currently had little.

I was startled out of my thoughts by a clap of thunder that rattled the roof. Within seconds, another clap of thunder, this time closer, shook the entire birthing house. Beads of rain struck the tin like pebbles. The interval between the drops shortened, working into a dull roar. Monique darted into the nearest room, and I heard the screech of iron on concrete as she shut down the window slats. Then she raced out, Basil hollering on her back. I ran into another room and slammed its window slats with a bang. The downpour ignited. The noise was deafening, as if herds of miniature beasts were crisscrossing at breakneck speed along the roof. I stared out the front door. Stray trees were pitched in battle with the wind, caught in a frenzied dance. Everything faded in and out of view behind sheets of water. The ground was a blur of ricocheting spray and dust in the throes of becoming mud. Monique ran up, slammed and bolted the door. Then we both ran to the wall farthest from the direction of the rain.

The wind came in waves, shaking the birthing house, threatening to break through the bricks. Rain drove through any open crack in the windows and leaked through the space around the closed front door. It blew in where the roof was not secured well. Dark water stains quickly spread down the walls and writhed across the uneven floor in what looked like tentacles. I gasped as I heard a loud, painful creak from the opposite end of the hall and saw the edge of the metal roof catch in the storm's fury and bend upwards. Taking advantage of this failing, the rain poured in. The sky was a blur the color of pavement.

"What a storm!" Monique yelled as she held Basil, covering him with her body and staring at the curled up roof. We huddled together, eyes wide, all senses on alert.

For over an hour I willed the roof to stay down as the storm churned outside. Then, as abruptly as it had come, it ended.

The damage was extensive. All the equipment was soaked. The old foam mattresses resembled giant sponges, weighing down the metal frames and streaming water. Wet papers stuck together, blue ink smudged and blurred, making ghostly sentences.

"We really must repair this building," I said.

"Yes. There is no question that it is not safe, even for consultations, while the rains are coming," she said.

We splashed through the large puddle around the door and opened it.

Already sunny again, the steam rose from the swollen ground littered with shattered palms, broken tree limbs, and straw roofs blown off homes and granaries. Countless muddy rivulets joined and split, all moving toward the sacred stream. I was accustomed to the stream being no more than a dried bed. Now it surged and flowed, cutting off the fields to the village's east. Its banks crumbled. What a trade. Life-giving rains came at the expense of devastating erosion; precious topsoil was washed away by the very thing needed to make it flourish. But for now, the world was refreshed, the oppressive heat dissipated. In the distance men readied their donkey carts for the fields, eager to plant their seeds.

Baby-weighing day came, and Mawa stood on the porch, a boy in each arm. She had been doing a pretty good job of bringing in the twins. They were an adorable eight months old, with their father's wide mouth and their mother's heart-shaped face. Lassiné's leather amulet swung around his naked waist as I weighed him. He was always a gram or two heavier than Fousseni. As I marked their weights on the charts, I noticed that, though they were still in the green healthy zone, the dots fell toward the yellow caution zone. I showed the pattern to Monique.

"Have they been sick?" she asked Mawa.

Mawa shook her head. Monique asked more questions and discerned that the twins had indeed been nursing well and that Mawa had been giving them supplemental water and food. However, she had been giving them well water, and not the cleaner pump water (complaining of its metallic taste), and she had been feeding them tŏ, rather than making special baby foods. Monique's advice: boil the well water if pump water isn't acceptable, and show up at baby food demonstrations.

Mawa nodded again as she leaned over, swung one son at a time belly down onto her back and cinched them tight. It was a good thing she was an ample woman; it was not going to get any easier carrying two growing children. Monique handed her back her charts.

"Good morning, Monique, Good morning, Fatumata," a man said as he walked onto the porch and into the clinic. "Sorry I am late."

It was Henri Traoré. A couple months back, in the stillness before the rains, he had expressed an interest in Monique's health work at the clinic. Henri was short and chunky as a cherub, with exceptionally full cheeks. He was not twenty and looked younger, but he could read and write. Monique was ecstatic when the dùgùtigi gave his nod of approval for Henri's participation. The plan was for him to be at the clinic two mornings a week, but with the rains he could only afford one for now. His presence gave me more time to weigh the babies and Monique more time to speak with the mothers.

The three of us worked all morning and into the afternoon. Many sick people came to the clinic. Villagers presented symptoms, such as fever, diarrhea, headaches, dizziness, a hacking cough, and Monique and Henri deciphered what the patients had and how to treat it. There were many infectious diseases: malaria, Hepatitis A or B, HIV, tuberculosis, amoebas, and other parasites. Not only were some of these diseases more prevalent during the rainy season (being water-related, such as malaria), but also people's immune systems were depressed from the lack of food before the new harvest, coupled with intense, long days in the fields. Fatigue also led to accidents, especially deep cuts to the feet and legs from ill-swung dàbas.

Henri measured pills and cleaned wounds as Monique and I concentrated on the mothers and babies. I ached from so much lifting and standing and grimaced as I stretched my neck and back. Henri, who was at the desk filling out the ledger, got up and offered his chair.

"Please stay," I said. "I'll get another one."

I took the tilty green chair from the corner of the room. I sat next to him and rested my head on my hand. It was late. Elise and Karamogo had yet to show, though I had reminded her again about the bra deal yesterday. Monique counted and organized vials in the cabinet. I scanned the ledger, taking note that the mothers' names covered more than a page.

"Henri, can I see that?"

I flipped back through the long, lined pages filled with women's names, baby's weights, and advice given, all in Monique's long, careful script. The trend was obvious. Eighteen women almost a year ago, twenty-three last spring, twenty-seven a couple of months ago. Today, over thirty.

At half past noon Monique went to the family compound and returned with rice and chicken sauce. She had told me Henri would be eating lunch with us and that he loved to eat. So, I had asked Louis to kill one of my many chickens for the meal. Henri consumed it all with relish and abandon, and left with a serene smile. Monique and I closed up and headed out to my house, where I wanted to show her my newly completed oven.

"Henri is a big help, Monique. When did he get trained as a health worker?"

"He doesn't have any training. He is learning from me, which is good, but he wants to get his certificate, like I have. He hopes the village will pay for him to be trained, like they paid for me. But for now, the village does not have the money."

"So, if Henri gets trained to work with you, will *he* have someone else pick up his salary, or will he have to give it to his father?"

Monique shrugged.

I knew the answer. I was being rhetorical out of frustration. Henri might be younger than Monique. He might be less experienced. But he was a man.

"I *am* going to talk to the dùgùtigi about your salary," I said.

"Ahh, Fatumata. Pati."

She glanced at me before looking down again at her shuffling feet. I sensed that she now was ready to talk about something else.

"What about Oumou?" I asked. "I can't believe that Soloman died. He was so giggly and cute when I saw him last month. He didn't seem sick to me."

"He was not sick. He got a serious cut, here." She pointed to her thigh. "It became infected. He died, all stiff like this," she made her neck and back rigid. "I have seen babies die this way, if the midwife does not sterilize the knife before cutting the cord. There are nuns who come out to Nampossela and give tetanus vaccinations, but Oumou missed their visits and Daouda did not want her to go into Koutiala for them."

"It would be so much easier if you could do the vaccinations yourself," I said.

"Yes, yes. That would be very, very good. But how can I, without a way to store them? I can't get a generator and refrigerator."

We arrived at my home and stood before the oven. It looked anything but new, constructed from a well-worn oil barrel. I had gotten the plans from the Peace Corps and had the local blacksmith put it together. He cut the rusted orange barrel in half, nestled one half inside the other, and left an air space all around like a giant thermos. He then cut a hinged door in one end and welded in a rack. The whole contraption lay on its side, covered in a good layer of mud for insulation and for keeping the powdered milk can chimney in place, two bricks above the ground so that wood could be placed underneath.

"Very, very nice," Monique said, and put her hands on her hips. "What will you make for me?"

"Mango bread, banana bread, and tonight, bread with tomatoes and cheese on it, which we call *pizza*."

My mouth watered at the thought. Monique's expression did not convey the same enthusiasm. I could find flour and yeast for the dough, tomatoes, garlic, and onion for the sauce, and I had dried basil and oregano that my parents had sent me. Granted, the cheese was cubes of processed

Vache Qui Rit, "Laughing Cow," from a store in Koutiala, but that hardly mattered to me after being deprived so long.

"What about birth control for Oumou?" I asked. It was time to broach this subject. "She could keep pills or condoms here. They don't need refrigeration."

Monique opened the oven door and peered inside at the blackness before closing it again. She then touched the lop-sided chimney and flicked the metal with her fingers. Ting, ting, ting. We went inside. Monique leaned against the doorway while I got the large bag of flour down from my shelf and began scooping out cupfuls for the dough.

"Condoms are good, but I don't think the villagers will use them. The men here do not like them. They say they cannot feel anything with those . . . those hats on," she said.

To my dismay, the small pile of flour began to move. Little white worms wriggled and squirmed. I grabbed my sifter (inherited from a former volunteer) and another bowl and exited to the porch with Monique behind me.

"The men know that *le SIDA*—AIDS—has found us here in Mali and have been told that wearing condoms will protect them against it, but still they do not seem to care. Many don't understand it, or don't believe it," she said.

Le SIDA. It had indeed arrived in Mali, I thought, as I dumped the flour into the sifter and watched the collection of worms move about on the screen as the flour fell into the clean bowl below. HIV entered through the transient border towns, where young Malian men gathered before heading to Senegal, Guinea, and the Ivory Coast seeking better wages. Seeking any wages. The worst was Sikasso, the largest town in southern Mali, near the borders with Burkina Faso and the Ivory Coast. I had read a recent study, which found that nine in ten sex workers in Sikasso were HIV positive. Men, married or not, were infected and brought the disease home when they returned to their villages. In most of Mali, there was little knowledge of HIV and there was no testing. An AIDS death would be attributed to something else. And the problem was not just protection during sex. Monique's work certainly put her at risk, but she had only a sporadic supply of rubber gloves. She washed her hands. What else could she do?

"Many women here still use the old ways to avoid pregnancy. Sometimes they work and sometimes they don't." Seeing my puzzled look, Monique added. "They stay away from having sex for a while. They try different herbs, plants to drink, or to put up there." She pointed below her abdomen.

I dumped the worms onto the ground.

"Of course, it does not keep the women from getting sicknesses, even if it does protect them from getting pregnant."

"Why don't more women take the pill?"

"Some women here, en brousse, do not want it. They wish to have many children. Many do not know about the pill. For those who do, it isn't easy to get. First the doctor must see them, in Koutiala. Then each month they must pick up their pack of pills at the pharmacy near the hospital. As you know, it is very difficult for women to travel and to find money, especially if their husbands are against it. And it is not looked upon well, the taking of the pill. If a woman takes the pill she keeps it secret, otherwise, people will think she is a *sunguruba*."

Monique pronounced the word quickly, as if she did not want it to linger on her breath too long for fear of it sticking. A prostitute.

"Uh-hum. Even so, the pill is the best," Monique went on, "as the man does not have to know about it. Do not tell le gars, but I do this for myself. Since Basil was six months old. I get it every month in Koutiala, when I get supplies for the clinic."

She sucked both her lips in, making her mouth look like a puckered crease. She was thinking hard.

"Perhaps the doctor would let me put women on the pill here, perhaps if they saw him once first and me after that. Then I could store them here and the women could get them when they came to see me."

I thought about birth and birth control, about Monique's work and her salary, as I walked to the dùgùtigi's house. I was nervous. He wanted to talk to me about the birthing house project; the village elders had met and had decided whether we could go ahead with plans for repairs. Besides discussing the fate of this building, I wanted to talk about Monique's salary and had no idea how he would respond. The dùgùtigi was kind and thought the world of Monique, yet I was asking for something that countered cultural norms. I didn't like putting him in an awkward situation, but saw no other choice.

I also wanted to inquire about John working, and maybe living, in Nampossela. The Peace Corps had recently decided not to replace John with another volunteer when he left next year; his village was too remote, becoming inaccessible with the rains. A water resources volunteer was desperately needed in this area, and repairing the two wells by the birthing house, part of the original plan, would be much easier if he lived closer. John struggled with the decision to finish his service in his village. He had good friends and his well work had been successful, but he was tired of the logistics tied to such an isolated place. John put in a request to be transferred to Koutiala and would find out in a few weeks whether the Peace Corps would honor it. If so, John would officially rent an apartment in Koutiala, but, in reality and unofficially, he would live here. I wanted to be sure the dùgùtigi was okay with that.

Just outside the compound entrance, I heard the rhythmic, dull thud of a pestle pounding grain. Mawa, the twins tied on her back, and a small girl were alternating thrusts into the hourglass shaped mortar. The gigantic vessel rocked towards the girl with every plunge from Mawa's pestle, threatening to crush her. But each time, the girl mustered everything she had, drove her smaller pestle into the grain, and kept the mortar in place. The muscles in their arms and backs flexed and moved in the perfectly timed dance of making flour.

Mawa stopped when she saw me, set the hefty tool against the wall and came across the small yard, scattering chickens and collecting small children along the way. By the time she reached me there were seven boys and girls standing behind her and peering out at me. The dùgùtigi was in the opposite corner of the compound, on a small rug of woven plastic strips. I could hear airy whispers of Arabic as he surrendered to the motion of his daily prayers, resting on his knees, then bending his head to the earth. Mawa motioned for a girl to get me their only seat, an old bamboo chair tied together with spotted strips of goat hide. Despite my insistence that I could sit on a mat, she put me in the chair in the center of the compound and then sat down herself on the mat beside me. I towered above her and the huddled children like an eager stalk of millet swaying above the rest of the crop.

The dùgùtigi finished after a few minutes and lowered himself down next to Mawa. Even when stools were available, they preferred sitting together, which I liked to see. He held his knees in his cracked, wide hands as one of his younger daughters nestled into his lap.

"My daughter, thank you for coming. I have held the village meeting and have spoken to the old men about your project to repair the birthing house. As you know the elders are responsible for guiding the village, respecting the laws that founded this village, and protecting this village from harm. In doing so, they believe that this project can only help; they have given their permission. They will work with the Association Villageoise to come up with part of the money, as you said, and to supply the workers, the donkey carts, and the bricks."

"Oh, that's great!" I slapped my hands together.

We discussed the details, of who would head the work of each quartier, of how soon I could get the money from USAID, and in what season the work could be completed. Gawssou, a friendly, quiet, and tireless man who had worked on my house, would help me organize the project. Though the work would not start until next spring, there was planning to be done.

"There is a possibility that Bakary might move here," I said, my left armpit perspiring, the first physical sign of my inner nervousness, "to Nampossela, if that is all right with you and the village. He could then do the well work for the birthing house project and train others to repair wells too."

"Very good. We will welcome him to Nampossela," he said. "Now I will have a daughter and a son from America."

He turned to Mawa and spoke in Minianka.

"*Akanyi, Fatumata, akanyi*—Good, Fatumata, good," her voice held reassurance in it.

"Dùgùtigi, I would like to talk to you about something else, too. It's about Monique and the salary she receives for her work."

He nodded.

"I have learned that Monique does not receive this money, that Louis takes it for her."

"Yes. What of it?"

Some of their kids were losing interest in me. One girl returned to the mortar and pestle. Two boys started playing.

"Well, I just think it's wrong. Louis takes the money, gives Monique a small part of it each month or sometimes nothing, and keeps the rest. Even though Monique worked for it. It's not fair to work and not get anything for it."

"Do you think I get paid for the work I do? No, no. Monique works for the family, so the family gets her money."

"But Monique works more than anyone I know!" I said, leaning toward him on the chair. "And it would be different if Monique received half the money, but she doesn't. The family suffers when she doesn't have the money to spend on them. Look at *petit* Karamogo, he's shrinking from malnutrition," I said, not really knowing if more money could help him. "Look at her house, it's so small and has no nyegen and no kitchen."

My knees lightly knocked together as I trembled with emotion.

"When it comes to this family, they have a particular situation," he said. "It was me who wanted Monique to take this work for the village. Louis did not wish it at first. It is the village that decided to give the money to Louis, and it is Adama, the village secretary, who is in charge of who signs for it. He has been schooled in how to do this, of how to work with money."

I had seen the dùgùtigi's hard, squared off fingers perform many tasks, from repairing woven straw mats, to pulling tufts of cotton from thorny plants, to hoeing and seeding an entire field. I could not imagine them holding a pencil or a pen. For that, he and the other elders of the village had to rely on others.

"Can't you talk to Adama? Or can't I?"

"No, he will not listen. It will not do anything."

Why did Adama have the right to decide? Was this just taking to the extreme the idea that women's work is not something you pay for?

"But you could talk to Monique's boss," he said.

"She has a boss?"

"Mr., uh, who is he?" he asked, circling his hand and encouraging his brain to release the name. "Uh, Mariko. Lassiné Mariko. He is the *patron*—the head of the health agents. He is at the hospital in Koutiala."

The bamboo chair creaked and swayed with relief as I rose to leave. Sensing the conversation was over, Mawa nodded and gave a small wave. The dùgùtigi got up, one joint at a time, and walked me to the entranceway.

"Good luck," he whispered.

The next time I went to Koutiala was not to see Mariko, but Pascal. John was in town and we had decided to visit Pascal's place of work: the prison. John, Monique, and I walked along the highway's steep berm as trucks and mopeds raced by, coating us in clouds of hot red dust. The prison was just north of the market, after the traffic circle, and not far from the Catholic church and the hospital.

It felt good to be out of the village, but we noticed a change. The checkpoints along the major road going in and out of Koutiala were bustling with *gendarmes* (policemen) in tan uniforms and green fatigues, almost all carrying guns. We were used to the armed soldiers examining an identity card every now and then and asking for an occasional bribe, but now they seemed to be stopping every car, truck, and moped that passed and demanding papers from the drivers and passengers.

The growing unrest in Bamako was having an effect. There were whispered desires for multiparty elections after decades of the UDPM, the United Democratic Party of Mali, General Traoré's party, being the sole choice on the ballot. Rumors of General Traoré's wife going on extravagant overseas shopping sprees reinforced the belief that Mali had corruption at the highest levels of the government. Even villagers knew that it wasn't just the general eating people's money. The dùgùtigi of Nampossela did not belong to the UDPM, whereas the chief of Sinsina, a neighboring village, did. The difference was noticeable. Nampossela's dùgùtigi had a mud brick home, no nyegen, and a small moped. The chief of Sinsina enjoyed a house made of fired bricks, a concrete latrine area, two separate houses for his wives, metal furniture, and a truck of his own. He was the area's UDPM representative, charged with the authority to collect money from the villages to "support the party."

Luckily, we walked past the checkpoint with a wave; we weren't on wheels, and besides, they knew the local Peace Corps volunteers. The entrance to the prison was like a castle. The outer gate led to a tall room, at the end of which was a second gate that opened onto the prison yard. Several guards stood by a table. One of them was Pascal.

Monique and Pascal walked close to each other and shared in private jokes. As always, John and I gave them their space; there were so few times when they could be together. The prison was a big open yard with a square building in the center. The walls went up two and a half stories, unadorned except for open cell doors. The prisoners were mostly men, about two hundred of them, clad not in uniforms, but in old, stained clothes, typical of what was worn for field work. They seemed well fed and were certainly friendly, shaking our hands and marveling at our Bambara. A few young women hung out by the doors of the building. Maybe they were prisoners, or were there to cook and provide for relatives, but their shorter skirts and their keeping to the shadows told me that they provided other services.

We lingered with Pascal into the late afternoon, until it was past time to head back to the village. We finally slipped through the outer gate and began our long walk back to Monique's parents' house and our motorcycles. Along the way, Monique grabbed John's and my arms and pointed across the street. There, covered in dust and brown rags, danced the crazy woman that I had seen when I first moved to Nampossela. She skipped and tripped along, thrusting her bony limbs in all directions, and occasionally yelling. Her matted, yellowed hair flopped about. She paid no heed to anybody or anything, only to an urge deep inside herself. The steady stream of people, carts, and mopeds flowed around her.

There were no social or medical programs here for the mentally ill. In the village, people with mental illness were cared for by their family, fed and kept clean, but this woman seemed to be on her own. I had asked the dùgùtigi about her. He, in turn, had consulted his *marabout* (Muslim mystic), who was able to divine her story. The crazy woman was from Chad. She had had a fiancé but was in love with another man. When the fiancé discovered that her heart did not belong to him, he had her cursed. From that time she had wandered aimlessly, never knowing who she was, from where she came, or where she was going. True or not, the moral of the story was evident: behold the fate of the unfaithful woman.

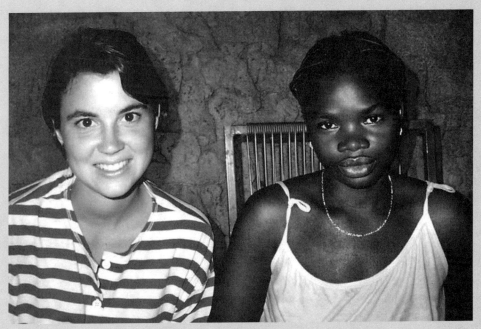

Kris Holloway and Monique Dembele

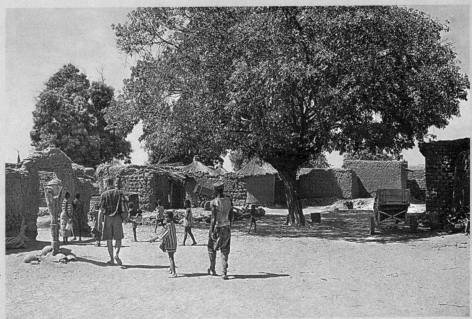

Village of Nampossela

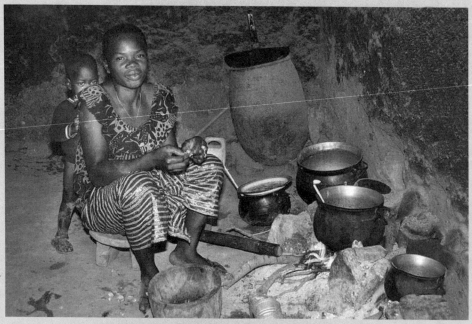

Bill Holloway

Monique prepares dinner while her son Basil hides behind her

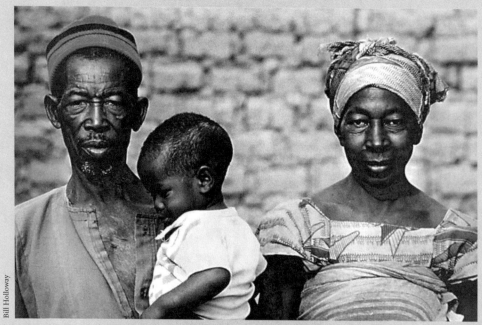

Bill Holloway

Louis and Blanche Dembele, Monique's in-laws, and their grandson Basil

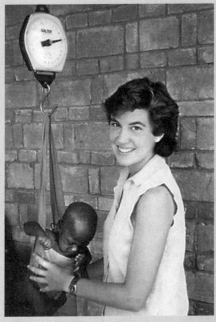

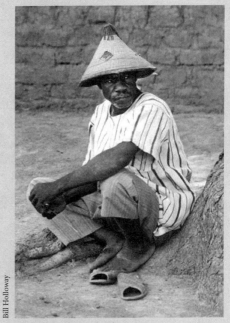

Bill Holloway

Kris weighing Fousseni Dembele at
Nampossela's health clinic

Bakary Dembele, the *dùgùtigi* (chief)
of Nampossela

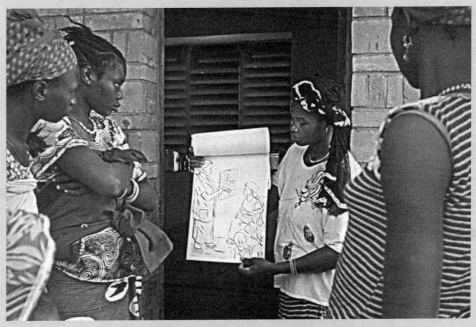

Monique conducting a health demonstration

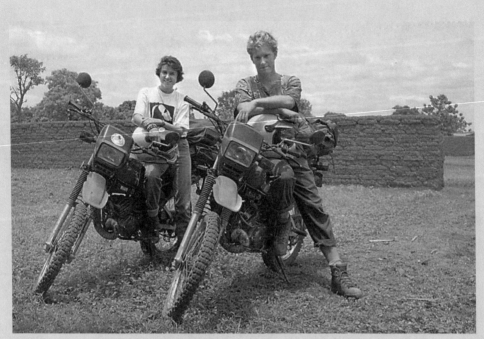

Kris with John Bidwell atop Yamaha 125s

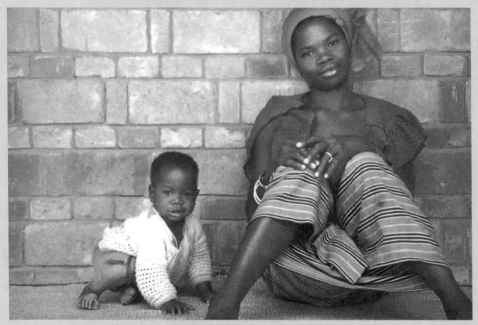

Basil and Monique

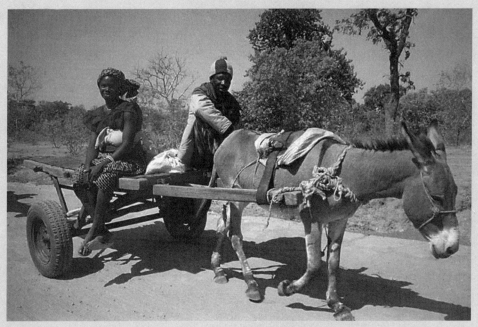

Monique traveling by donkey cart

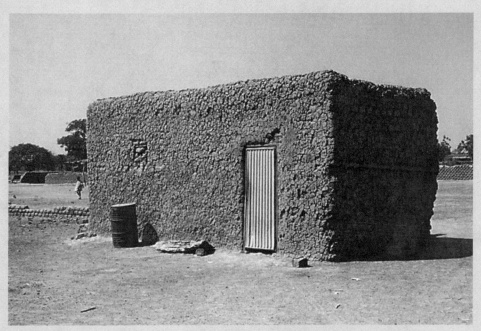

Monique and François' house

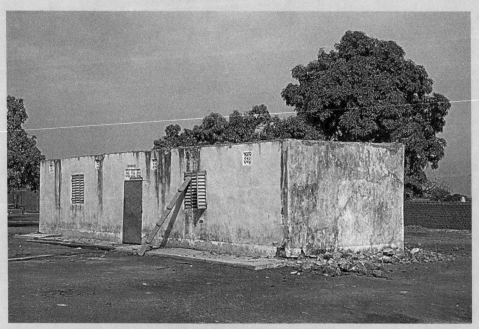

Nampossela's birthing house under repair

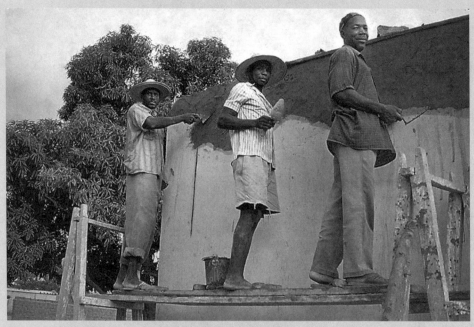

Three masons putting an outer layer of cement on the birthing house

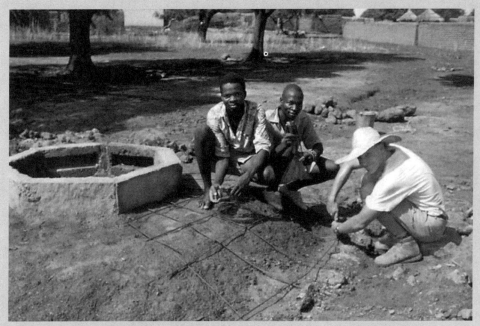

John and apprentices rebuilding birthing house well

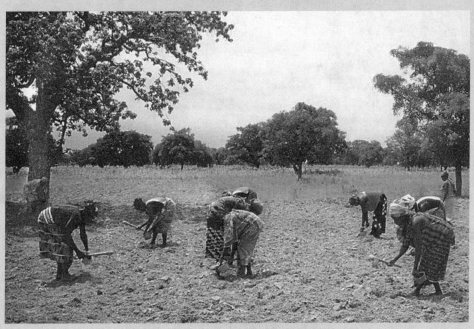

Women planting a communal field of beans and peanuts

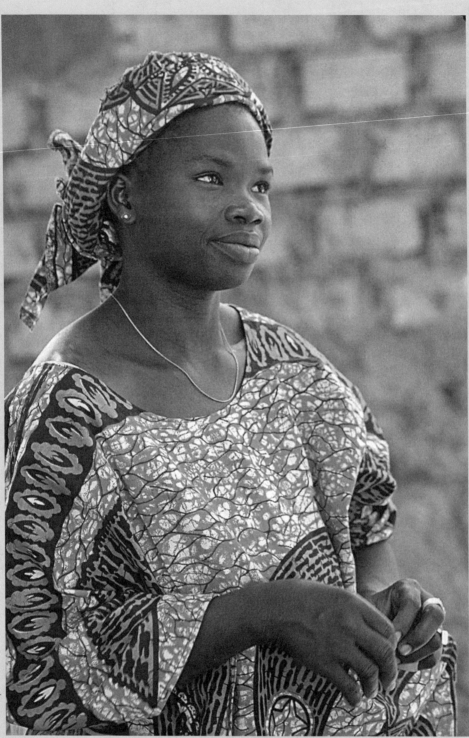

Bill Holloway

Monique

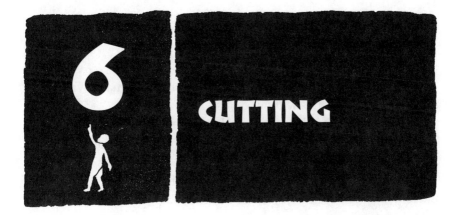

6

CUTTING

I REMOVED MY HELMET, PLACED IT ON THE HANDLEBARS, AND EXAMINED MYSELF IN THE MOTORCYCLE'S REARVIEW MIRROR. My hair was a concert of split ends and my face was edged with dirt. I was hardly presentable, but it would have to do. I looked out across the old colonial buildings that made up the Koutiala hospital and maternity ward: long, faded yellow structures with rows and rows of rooms spilling out onto communal porches. Up close, the complex of buildings was even more dismal. Small, dusty banana bushes dotted the area, and scattered windblown medical trash—soaked dressings, needles, and gloves—was piled up in corners. I ascended the steps and stood on the immense veranda; green iron doors linked the rooms in a line like railroad cars. I wondered through which one of them I might find Mr. Mariko.

Two patients walked ghostlike through the rooms, their skeletal profiles appearing in doorways and windows and disappearing again. Monique had said that tuberculosis, syphilis, and AIDS brought most of them here and ensured they never left. Family members sometimes moved onto the hospital grounds to help care for their dying relatives.

Finally, I spotted a man in a white coat and asked him where I could find Mr. Mariko. He led me into the building, through rooms of empty beds and dirty floors, until we entered a long hallway with doors on both sides. He pointed to the fourth door on the left.

A square-faced man with bushy eyebrows sat behind a metal desk, writing.

"Good morning," I said.

"Good morning," he responded, standing up and smoothing the sitting-induced creases on his brown suit pants.

"Mr. Lassiné Mariko?"

"Yes," he smiled, leaned over the desk and shook my hand with a firm grip. Perfect teeth. Palms without calluses.

"I am Fatumata Dembele. I live in Nampossela and work with Monique Dembele, the midwife there. I attended a training with her on infant food demonstrations and met you then."

"Oh, yes, yes. I remember. Please sit down," he pointed to a metal chair and folded his hands in front of him on the desk. "What can I do for you?"

I told him.

"*Ce n'est pas normal, non*—It is not normal, no," he said. "I will come out to Nampossela and speak with the family. Is that all, Fatumata?"

"Yes, but, what day can I tell them you'll come?"

"Oh, I don't know. I am very busy. But I will come out soon, yes, very soon." He stood up briskly. "Now, I must get back to work."

We said our good-byes and I left, relieved that the meeting had gone smoothly.

Basil sat on the ground, feet spread out in front of him, eating a section of orange. Dark, shiny lines of spilled juice ran over and down his ample, dusty belly. To his left, Monique, Blanche, and Elise went about the business of transforming *karité* nuts (shea nuts) into oil. They had already gathered the large, buckeye-shaped tree nuts, tossed out the rotten ones, roasted them, pounded open their hard shells in a mortar, and now, in the fading light of day, were grinding them.

The three women knelt on the ground, each with a large flat rock held steady between her knees and another smaller flat rock gripped in both hands. In quick, strong strokes, they pressed their entire weight upon their outstretched arms. The nuts became thick maroon paste that pooled in the sand. As the women rocked to and fro, Blanche's flat withered breasts beat against her naked torso while Karamogo's head lolled back and forth on Elise's back. Blanche chattered away. Elise piped up every now and then. Monique said nothing. She had been quiet all evening. Louis was asleep on the bamboo recliner by his hut. François was gone. In fact, he had not returned for dinner at all.

I had been an onlooker since dinner's end. Monique had let me try grinding for twenty seconds before nodding her thanks and taking back her rock. She was either protecting me from such laborious work or protecting the smooth uniform pool of oil from my coarse contributions. I wasn't sure which. It had been several days since John and I had eaten dinner with the family. Since his move to the village a week ago, we had spent twenty-four hours a day together and had eaten most of our dinners at my house. A meal at my house didn't mean a meal alone anymore. We were relishing speaking English together, eating Western food (John had brought dried taco seasonings, beans, and glory of all glories, Pop Tarts) on plates, with forks, and being together without another good-bye lurking just ahead.

"Aw ni su," came greetings from the compound entrance.

"Aw ni su," said Louis, quickly sitting up.

John and Gawssou appeared. Gawssou had become a permanent fixture at John's side whenever he was out in the village. Though Gawssou spoke no French and John could barely get by in Bambara, they had somehow connected. Gawssou was constantly pushing his large blue knit cap back up his forehead. Specter thin, always hungry, always quick to laugh, he was, as I was coming to learn, one of Nampossela's hardest workers.

They greeted everyone, then sat down by me.

"Gawssou and I have figured out what each quartier will need to supply in terms of bricks and manpower if the maternity ward project is funded." John said. "I think we'll also be able to repair the nearby wells. The dùgù-tigi says everyone's very excited."

We had written a grant to USAID for $3,000 US. If they funded it, the village would have to supply the equivalent of $1,000 worth of manpower. This included the gathering and transportation of bricks, sand, and gravel, and the mason work.

"Great," I said. Then I asked Gawssou in Bambara, "Each quartier has agreed to do the work?"

"Yes," he said. "But we will see if the Konés do their share of the work or not."

The Konés were known for their relaxed work ethic.

"It is the Koulibalys that are the lazy ones," John said, turning to Gawssou. Gawssou was a Koulibaly, the joking cousins of the Keitas, and John was a Keita. "They do nothing but eat beans."

"Ah, no!" Gawssou cackled, the long vertical facial scars along his cheekbones bending as he grinned. He straightened up and leaned closer toward John. "We have no beans; it is you who eat the beans."

"You eat so many beans, they can hear your gas all the way to Segou," John said, an endearing line I had heard at least once a day since his arrival. His hand flew into the air and pointed north to the distant city.

At this, Louis, Blanche, Elise, and Gawssou all broke out in laughter.

"Eh, Bakary!" Gawssou said, grabbing John's arm.

Monique managed a brief smile and returned to her work. Something was wrong. She always laughed at John's jokes.

"*Bon*," she grunted and finished a last stroke with the stone and sat back on her heels. The pile of karité nuts was gone. Tomorrow they would boil the paste, transforming it into a thick creamy butter that looked like yellowed Crisco. In the kitchen it was used in sauces and for frying, contributing a rich nutty taste that I loved, but it was also the main ingredient in soap and a common lamp fuel.

"Gawssou, will you eat something?" Monique asked.

Gawssou nodded, adjusting his cap.

"Bakary? More tŏ?"

"No thanks, Monique. I stuffed myself with your tŏ at dinner. Best tŏ in Mali."

I followed her into the cooking hut.

"Fatumata, give me those little pieces of firewood," she ordered, pointing to a small pile jumbled outside the door.

I handed her the sticks. She began reheating the sauce.

"Monique, is something wrong?"

She took a deep breath and stirred the sauce vigorously.

"Le gars was out with someone else again."

"Like he has done before . . ."

"No!" she almost yelled, then in a quieter voice said, "No, he has not done *this* before. Yes, I have brought out food to him, in another compound. Yes, he has eaten it with his girlfriend. But this time, did you not notice how weak the sauce was tonight? I have nothing left with which to buy meat or vegetables. Only a few onions from his tiny garden. For three days, we have lived on onions. And, I saw her! She was wearing new clothes. New clothes! Do you know whose money bought these clothes? Eh? She has new clothes while we have water for sauce."

"Monique, if . . ."

"I am not finished telling you the rest of it," she interrupted. She whipped the small pot of sauce into froth with her steel, slatted spoon. "Pascal. He told me that he is on reserve with the African Peace-Keeping Forces. He has been put on alert and could be sent anywhere. Maybe far from here." As she said this, her words and emotions foamed out. Gradually her stirring slowed and she shook her head once, emphatically, as if it was the final gesture needed to clear her head.

"Fatumata, *haketo*—excuse me. You must be so tired of listening to these problems with no end."

"Monique, I am not tired of listening to your problems."

I leaned against the wall, as she poured the hot sauce for Gawssou into a small bowl, and placed it on top of a bowl of tŏ (always prepared for the unexpected guest and eaten cold the next morning if one didn't show up). Then it dawned on me. François' squandering of resources didn't seem to bother anyone in the family but her, and Pascal's presence in her life was secret. I hadn't been around this week, especially in the evening, and we hadn't talked alone since John arrived. I was used to depending on Monique, and now I saw that she, too, had come to depend on me.

Weeks later, Mariko still had not come, but he *had* talked to Monique in Koutiala and asked her to tell Adama to hand over her salary. Not what was needed. Monique took it in stride, telling *me* to be a little more patient. I was fidgety and I wanted to talk with Mariko again. One morning, I decided it was time and went to the clinic early to see if Monique needed anything at the market while I was in Koutiala.

As I hopped onto the clinic porch, I found Henri inside, but no Monique.

"She is at the maternity ward," Henri said. "She told me to tell you when you arrived to join her there. It is your friend Korotun who has requested you."

I raced to the maternity ward. Though it had not weathered the rainy season well, at least women could still give birth there.

I knew Monique was worried about Korotun having strength enough to push the baby out, but I was filled with hope at the thought that Korotun was finally having her long-awaited child. I was glad that I could help at her birth. Monique had taught me the details of birth: what a mucous plug was and what it means to lose it, how the tiny donut-shaped cervix dilates ten times its normal size, and the importance of the glorious placenta. And I had seen many times the miracle of what a woman's body could do.

Korotun lay naked on the slab, knees up, and head against the wall at an uncomfortable angle, her chin on her chest and her mouth slack. Monique was next to her, quiet. They were motionless, resting; only the pungent smell of impending birth moved through the room.

"How far has she dilated, Monique?" I asked in a soft voice, wondering how close Korotun was to completing the first stage of labor, the opening of the cervix, the womb's door.

"She is almost done; it is almost time to start pushing."

Pushing was the second stage of labor. After gently cradling the fetus for nine months, the woman's uterine muscles had to move the baby through the cervix, along the birth canal of the vagina, and out to the world. The third and final stage was the expulsion of the placenta.

"Korotun, it's me. Fatumata."

I searched her tense face. She seemed far away, as if her spirit had drifted beyond the horizon.

"Fatumata," she blurted and her eyes opened wide. She grabbed my hand. "Fa . . ."

She was cut off by a contraction. Her body was no longer hers; she had to submit to its will. Everything was secondary to the push. She grimaced and groaned, her belly looked as hard as concrete for a moment, and then she released.

"I am so tired," she panted, "I cannot do this."

"You can do it, Koro," Monique said. "You can."

Monique shot me a nervous glance.

"Let's get you sitting up, where you can push with more strength."

"No, no. I can't." Korotun said and flopped her head from side to side, rhythmic and delirious.

"I just want to rest, I just want to lay here. Please let me lay here."

Monique and I slowly raised her by the elbows. Unlike other women, there was nothing meaty about Korotun. Her ribs and backbone protruded, her skin too thin a canvas stretched over a meager frame. I felt the need to comfort her and snatched her clothes off the table, putting them between her bones and the wall. As we eased her back, she braced herself against the wall for another contraction. Her legs and neck muscles tightened. Her hold on my hand crushed my fingers. I pushed back as she leaned heavily into my arm. Monique stood across from me on the other side of Korotun, talking her through each contraction, reminding her to breathe. Monique and I guided her, letting the contractions build, gauging when they were cresting, and ordering her to push.

The hours passed. The room grew hot, wet, fertile.

"The baby is coming down," Monique said, wiping her brow. "It is working. You are doing it. Don't give up now."

"Good," I said. "I can see the baby's head."

Korotun nodded, panting, eyes closed to mere lines, deeply etched crows' feet shooting off in rays.

"It is time now," Monique said in a directive tone. "On this next one I want you to push with all your strength."

She pressed down. The head pushed forward, and then finally burst out in a spray of blood.

"Good, Koro," Monique said. "Now stop, stop. Just breathe."

Monique held the head in her palms, investigating with her fingers and thumb to make sure that the umbilical cord was not around the neck.

The head hung there, streaked with white vernix and crimson blood, between Korotun's splattered thighs. She panted and seemed unable to release my hand. There was so much blood. I looked at Monique, gauging her alarm, but she remained focused on Korotun.

"On this next one, push slowly," Monique said.

Korotun pushed the shoulders out and the rest of the being quickly surrendered to the world. What a big baby. Monique quickly put the crying newborn on Korotun's chest while I wrapped clean pagnes around it. The baby looked fine, but there was so much blood. Monique quickly took another pagne and pressed it between Korotun's legs. She held it in place with one hand and checked the cord, still hanging out, with the other. The small medicine trunk was open. On top was a syringe of Pitocin, in case of a severe hemorrhage. If that failed to work, a woman was balanced on the back of a moped, like a goat condemned for market, and raced to the Koutiala hospital. Please don't let what happened to Bintou happen to Korotun, I begged.

Monique focused on the pagne, the wet, glistening red soaking one side. We watched and waited while the baby's cries pierced the air around us.

"Is it a boy?" Korotun managed in a husky whisper.

Monique didn't answer, but remained fixed on the amount of blood that was reaching her hands. Slowly, she lifted the pagne, gave a sigh of relief, and left the cloth to rest in place. Then Monique took the wailing baby off Korotun's chest and unwrapped the cloth to answer her question.

Korotun took one look at her daughter and rolled her head away from us.

I peeked down at the pinkish-white face. She had Korotun's full pink lips, Dramane's straight nose, and almond eyes. I knew they would make a gorgeous child. Monique listened to the baby's heart and breathing, moved the legs up and down, and tested reflexes by inserting her index finger into the palm of each tiny, grasping hand. The baby yelled more, her face reddened and wrinkled. Monique quickly wrapped her back up, quieting the piercing cries, and put her back down.

"She quiets easily," Monique said. "Unlike her mother."

She walked over to her ledger and pen on the windowsill.

"Put her to the breast, it will help your placenta come out."

Korotun complied.

"She is so beautiful," I said.

"Is she beautiful? To you perhaps. She would be beautiful in her father's eyes if she were a son."

Korotun's daughter took quickly to her mother's breast. For the first day or two Korotun's body would provide thick, antibody-dense colostrum before the milk came in. Korotun groaned as a contraction rippled through her. Time for the placenta. As Monique removed the blood-soaked pagne, something did not look right. Usually, I did not peer so intently between a woman's legs, but Korotun was the first friend I had seen give birth and I dropped my usual attempts at guarding privacy.

The right side of her vagina was shredded as if the birth had been literally ripped from her. Her vagina looked less like an organ of wonder than a hideous wound. I involuntarily cringed and turned toward the slatted window. Since working more closely with Monique, I had glimpsed women's vulvas that were distorted and uneven, some with jagged edges, conditions I attributed to the young age of most mothers and to the process of birth, but I had never seen anything like this. I cleared my throat and turned back around.

Monique examined the placenta as if she was looking over a piece of meat at the market. After determining that it was intact and that nothing was left inside, she dropped it into a plastic tub (it would later be buried in Korotun and Dramane's compound) and cut the cord, freeing the baby. Korotun lay still on the slab, eyes closed, arm around her sucking daughter. Monique began washing off Korotun with soap and water, cleaning the entire region around her vagina. Then she got her flashlight, a needle and thread and examined what she needed to sew back together. I began cleaning up, moving the afterbirth tub, and washing down the few hard surfaces that were Monique's workspace. When Monique was finished, we helped Korotun get to her feet. She was shaky, even with our support.

"Now I must go home," Korotun said, bundling the infant and starting to strap the newborn to her back.

"Hey, hey. What is this?" Monique said in an exasperated voice. She took back the baby. "You can rest here. Your work can wait."

"At least let me rest at my house."

Monique glared at her.

"Lie down in the other room until we have finished cleaning up. Then we will bring you to your home where you can bathe."

Korotun relented. She had no energy to fight. We settled her and the baby in the other room. Monique wiped and scrubbed, more slowly than usual. We looked in on them every ten minutes or so, and after an hour Monique gave her a more thorough check up. Monique pressed lightly on Korotun's stomach and took her blood pressure. The two of them had another exchange of words, the result being Korotun resting another half-hour before we hoisted her from the bed to take her home. It was hard for me to see this as enough rest. She had suffered labor, lost blood, and her recovery period was just over an hour on a tattered foam mattress placed over a sagging rusty bed frame.

Korotun insisted on carrying the baby on her back, even though she needed us to prop her up from either side. Monique swung open the front door and the noon light hit us like the glare of snow on a clear winter day, rendered us sightless and still. I shielded my eyes and looked down as we began walking out. Soon I noticed a rivulet of blood flowing down

Korotun's right leg, curving behind her calf, behind the ball of her ankle, and under her foot. The back of her flip-flop was red-brown and wet. Every now and then her heel slipped a little on the blood, leaving a trail of dark waning moons behind us.

Dramane was not at home, but his aunt and cousin were. We poured Korotun a bucket bath and placed it in the nyegen, while they looked on with concern. Monique explained to them how hard the birth was for her and that she needed to recuperate. After extracting promises from Korotun not to work and reminding her that we would be checking in, we left for the clinic.

"She is so hard-headed," Monique said, on our return. "We must watch her. I'll go back in a few hours, to make sure she isn't working."

"Why does she want to go home so quickly?"

"She will try and please Dramane. She will cook a good sauce and make a clean home, hoping he will notice less the absence of a son. The baby was big for her to push out. She tore badly, and it will take a while to get better. She will need to keep herself clean. But her uterus is firm, back to size."

For a demonstration, or for emphasis, she held up her hand and brought the fingers together into a fist. A tight uterus was a healing uterus.

"What tore so badly?"

"The opening. It could have been much worse, since she is so small and it is her first baby. Almost every woman rips on her first baby. Have you not noticed?"

Ripping was such a horribly accurate word.

"I've noticed that women seem to tear when the baby's head comes out. But I can't tell what's tearing and what's coming out from the womb with the baby."

"The womb's blood is dark, while a rip's blood is bright red. Perhaps you have not seen this yet, but some women tear back through to their bottoms." Monique traced a curved line in the air. "The big problem comes afterward. If they do not get stitched up and do not keep clean, pati, the infections I have seen . . ."

She shook her head and wrists.

"That must hurt," I said with a grimace.

"It hurts. Most women have not known this pain since they were young; since their *koloboli*," Monique said, scrunching up her face and thinking, "What is it called in French? . . . Oh, yes, I think it is called *l'excision*. The excision."

I wracked my brain. I remembered reading about female circumcision in a Peace Corps manual; it was a ritual that entailed the clipping of the clitoral hood. What I had seen at the birthing house seemed far worse.

"Excision?" I asked.

"You don't know of it?"

"No," I shook my head.

"You have not had it done? You have not been cut?" Monique looked concerned.

"No," I said, and reluctantly added, "tell me what you mean by 'cut.'"

Monique paused, choosing her words carefully.

"Well, here, it is done when girls are nine, or ten, like that. It is hard for me to remember exactly when it was done. It was so long ago. I was in Koutiala, in a small, closed hut with my friends and other girls I knew, other girls my age. I remember being very excited that it was time. I remember being talked to, being held down tightly, being held very still, and . . . Hup! The old woman sliced."

Monique dropped her hand. I jumped.

"It was so fast, it happened before I knew it. There was so much blood, but none of us cried. But afterwards, pati . . . we cried. Oh, we cried! When they would clean us, we had to stay still, with our legs apart, to prevent infection. They cleaned us with alcohol. Ah! I have never had such pain. Never, even in childbirth."

She looked at me as if to say, "Now you remember, right?"

I shook my head, eyes frozen open.

"You really haven't had it done."

"No. But, what exactly did they cut on you?"

"I don't know, some parts that we didn't need. All I know is that it took a long time to heal, a long time to go to the nyegen without it hurting."

My stomach felt empty and my feet did not want to move. I thought back on the births I had assisted. The vulva and vagina had appeared to be merged. Sometimes the opening was thin, notched, and scarlike. It was not supple as I imagined it should be; yet I didn't know what a woman's vagina should look like during birth.

"Who cut you?"

"An old woman in Koutiala. She is dead now. It is the old women who do this work. You have met the one in Nampossela; you know her, the old Korotun, Korotun Dembele. We visited her once, in a hamlet. She was the big one."

I remembercd her. She was big in a dilapidated way. Her large head housed watery eyes, and her once mighty arms dangled in great bags from her bones. I sat beside her, gave her kola nuts, and drank millet beer out of her calabash. I shook her right hand, unaware that it had carved out girl's genitals for a living. Tears welled in my eyes as I thought of Monique, and of her mother, Jeanne, before her, and her daughter, Gené, after her, all under the knife.

"She used no anesthesia?" I asked.

Monique shook her head and waited before she spoke again.

"I have never met a woman like you, who has not gone through koloboli. I thought every woman had it," Monique said, with that concerned, sad voice again. "Does anyone have it done in your country?"

"In the U.S.? No! I don't think so. There are people who circumcise boys, like you did with Basil, but no one that removes parts from girls."

"Hmmm. Here we say that koloboli helps girls become good wives and bear children. But, I can tell you, Fatumata, that I have noticed myself, that it does not help the baby pass through. As a midwife, I have certainly noticed this."

With that, we began walking again, side by side.

"*Maintenant*—Now—Mawa," Monique said, holding a flattened metal spoon in one hand and a plastic bag of black-eyed peas in the other, "listen closely and I will show you how to make baby food."

She sat next to a small fire with a bulbous pot of boiling water balanced on three large rocks. Mawa sat on a mat beside her with the twins as well as three other children. She sat close enough to the pot to watch, but kept a respectable distance. Small children had a horrible habit of stumbling into open fires.

Fousseni and Lassiné, at almost a year old now, could barely sit up. Their eyes were half-lidded and crusty, and they leaned their wasted little bodies, bare except for protective amulets on their waists, into Mawa. They may have been a miracle, but now they were dying. I saw it in their lethargy, pale complexions, and lackluster attempts at eating food. Their weights had slowly and steadily dropped for several months, taking a sharp turn downward in the last few weeks. It had happened so fast.

I couldn't help but contrast them to Basil who at a year and a half was storming about and had just cornered a chick. He was chunky and feisty. I was astonished that Monique could still lug his ample girth, but many women here carried their kids even at 20 kilos, over 40 pounds. I had carried Basil on my back only once, from the clinic to my house amid Monique's howling laughter, a distance long enough to make my back ache from the weight and my breasts sting from the pressure of the tied cloth. Since Basil had learned to walk, though, he preferred spending more time on his own feet, overturning bowls, and keeping livestock on the move.

The chick's kin were distraught. Its mother clucked and pattered to and fro, followed by her other offspring, all fluster and peeps. The hen issued some quick instructions; the trapped chick feigned left, skittered to the right and past Basil. The chicken clan made for the courtyard entrance and the relative safety of the village paths. Basil fell back on his wide naked bottom and hollered his disappointment. Monique ignored him. He got back up and, wailing all the way, ran into her lap. She put aside her spoon for a moment to position him at her breast.

"First, take these beans, Mawa, and grind them into a powder," Monique said, "this makes them easier to swallow since Fousseni and Lassiné do not yet have all their teeth."

Mawa got up, put one of the twins on her back, lay the other on the ground, and walked over to a large flat rock in the middle of the compound. She began to grind the beans expertly, like I had seen Monique do so many times with peanuts and karité nuts. Soon she had a pile of course bean flour.

We had done this same demonstration just a couple of weeks back for a large group of mothers. Mawa hadn't been there, but Elise had. We had yet to see Elise institute anything she may have learned. Karamogo remained the poster child for childhood sickness. I hoped with Mawa and the twins it would be different.

Sickness could come in an instant. Death was skulking behind every calabash of dirty water, untreated burn, or mosquito bite. This was true for anyone, but with their young immune systems, the children, after being weaned from protective breast milk, were especially vulnerable. Lack of the right foods during and after weaning was most important. Typically, a child's diet abruptly changed with the advent of a younger sibling. While the newborn got the bosom, the older child went straight from breast milk to adult food, with sips of well water. The toddler's digestive system had little time to adjust, and tõ with sauce did not have the concentration of vitamins and protein he or she needed. Even in lean times, I had learned, the men ate first, meaning that they skimmed the meat and vegetables before the remnants were passed on. Infectious diseases, mostly caused by drinking dirty water, took lives as well. The making of baby food, a new concept to the village women, tackled both these problems. It was high-protein food cooked in clean water.

"The dùgùtigi has five children with Mawa and three children with his other wife," Monique said, watching the twin on the ground by Mawa. "And he is looking to take yet another wife. If he wants all these children, he must feed them. If we succeed in bringing the pill to the village, he might let his wives use it as well."

"Mawa must make the baby food for a week or two, until she can see her babies are healthier. She must make it every day. Every day. This will be difficult, as I do not have the time to come here and do it."

Monique's schedule kept getting busier. We hadn't had a night in Koutiala with Pascal for weeks. Henri was a help, but he could not yet run the clinic on his own.

"I'll work with Mawa," I said.

My mind wandered. John was in the capital, awaiting word on the funding of our maternity ward project. I was worried about him, as the political situation in Bamako had worsened. Unlicensed vendors (forced by General Traoré to close down their shops) and students had demonstrated in Bamako by throwing rocks, looting stores, and burning automobiles. General Traoré had cracked down with an iron fist of teargas and mass arrests. Thousands had then taken to the streets to demand the dictator's resignation. I hoped John would return safely, and with good news about the funding.

I looked around the compound, with its scattering of pots, stones, mortars, and sigilans (small seats). The firewood, a jumble of twirling branches and asymmetric logs, was piled in a far corner. Mawa and her older daughters walked several kilometers into the bush to gather it. Draped over the pile was clean, wet laundry. The drying cloths were drawn taut between the branches and looked like outstretched bat wings.

One of the little girls who had been sitting by the fire got up and walked toward the woodpile. She squeezed in by the wall, squatted and strained and, after a minute, got up and walked away. Flies wasted no time settling onto the small mound left behind, the same flies that would soon gather on the bean powder, on the rim of the cooking pot, and on the tiny hands and faces of the twins. Normally, Mawa or an older daughter would sprinkle dirt on the pile, slide it onto a piece of cardboard and deposit it outside the compound door, or use a small cup, as Monique did for Basil, but this time, no one seemed to notice.

Mawa finished crushing the beans into a coarse powder, no lumps or shells to be found. She lifted the pagne, folded it to make a spout, and poured the powder into a small tin bowl.

"Good," Monique said, in her teacher's voice, directed, praising, expecting the best. "Now, we put three handfuls of powder into the water."

"Stir it until it thickens, like a sauce." She handed Mawa the spoon, "almost like the consistency of hot tŏ."

Mawa approached the pot, stirred it from her side, and spoke to Monique in Minianka.

"Fatumata," Monique said, "Mawa has an idea. And I think it is a good one. She said it is difficult to get beans and peanuts this time of year. That it will be difficult for women to use peanuts for baby food and not for the family sauce. That perhaps, if the village agrees, and if the women wish it, each family could bring a few beans and peanuts to plant, in a field, together."

"A communal field? Just for growing baby food?"

"Yes."

"What a great idea, Mawa, *a kanyi, i hakili kadi,*" I said, expressing my enthusiasm for the idea.

"*Aw ni ce,*" a husky voice greeted us. Korotun appeared in the compound doorway.

She shuffled across the yard. She had lost weight since the birth. Her cheeks were hollowed bowls and her skin was sallow. I could not tell if the yellowed shadow under her eyes was lack of sleep, lack of nutrition, or healing flesh.

"How are you? How's little Ami?" I asked.

"I have come for aspirin," she said listlessly, not lifting her gaze from the ground. She turned sideways so I could see her daughter bound to her back. Little Ami was as cute as the day she was born, with a symmetrical face, trim features, and lips that curved into a natural smile. Red threads hung delicately from her freshly pierced ears.

Monique strapped a now sleepy Basil onto her back, opened her bag, counted out two aspirin, walked to Korotun, and placed them in her open palm. She uttered small thanks and turned to go. Monique blocked her exit.

"Korotun, new mother, where are you going?" Monique said. "Are you so busy that you must take your aspirin and run?"

Monique smiled at her, trying to ignite some spark of the familiar in our friend.

"I can't today," she said and brushed past Monique. Her eyes were still and cold.

"Hey, the first months with a baby are not easy. Stay a while with us."

Her sentence was phrased politely, but was also an unmistakable command. Korotun did not look back, but drifted out.

"Something's wrong," Monique said, tightening her pagne and taking a bunch of tiny ripe bananas and a plastic bag of salt out of her bag and placing them on the ground. "Fatumata, can you finish with Mawa?"

"Yes," I said and watched Monique disappear after Korotun. *Please let it be anything but Dramane,* I thought to myself. I turned back to concentrate on Mawa, who was still stirring the pot.

"Maintenant, we will cut up the bananas, and add them." I tore off two bananas, peeled them, and dropped them in. Mawa, arms now cradling the twins, did the same.

"Now we put in two fingers of salt," I said, adding a pinch. "Voilà."

Mawa said something in Minianka, which I thought indicated the porridge was done.

"How does it taste? It looks . . . ah . . . good," I said, looking at the thick brownish goo.

Mawa dipped her finger in, put it to her mouth, and nodded. She dipped it in again, blew on her finger and thrust it into Lassiné's mouth. He frowned, his first expression since my arrival, and spat it out. A fly landed on a glob of food stuck on his bottom lip. Mawa then swung Fousseni off her back and into her lap to give him a try. He was no more impressed with the menu than was his brother. She continued balancing them in her lap, dipping her fingers, blowing, and feeding them while they pushed the food back out of their mouths with their tongues. My mother always said that a child would eat anything if he was hungry enough, but now I had my doubts.

"Little by little they will learn to eat it," I said, trying to sound confident. "Now Mawa, you can take bean flour or peanut flour to make this, and add any kind of fruit: mango, papaya, guava. When they are a little older and are used to eating this food, we will add *sunbala* and leaves."

Sunbala is ground-up néré tree nuts used to flavor sauces and is rich in vitamins and minerals.

"The water must boil before you add the flour. Try and get water from the pump, it's cleaner than the well water. Make the porridge for them twice a day. I know it's hard to do, but it's the only way they'll get their strength back."

Mawa clicked her tongue in understanding.

"I'll be back tomorrow," I said, "to make another porridge with you."

Neither of the twins had eaten much. Lassiné was falling asleep and Mawa covered his face with a light cloth to keep the flies away. Fousseni stared at the wall, managing enough energy to fend off his mother's occasional attempts at feeding. For now, we needed to concentrate on getting food into the boys, but I realized that we needed to tackle sanitation issues as well. Mawa must cover her food, the kids must use a nyegen, and everyone needed to wash their hands with soap. If I had learned one thing from my year in Nampossela, it was that the most mundane habits could separate life from death.

Late that evening, the thud of beating drums drew me into the Koulibaly section of town. An elder was dead, an elder who had belonged to the *Koori*. Louis had told me about this secret society of men, of which he had once been a member. Every three years, a new group of young men (not women, and not men who were previously Christian or Muslim) were initiated. This rite involved the sacrifice of goats and a dance with fire, during which the members sang "those who know, say the fire is water to drink." The Koori was also said to bring the rain. Every June, the men circled the village three times, drank dòlo, and made sacrifices in the small grove next to my house, where I occasionally heard voices and rustlings.

When a member of the Koori died, a sacrifice and the fire dance were necessary as well.

As I approached the central meeting space, I could see the tree branches and leaves above the huts dancing with shadows thrown by torches and shaking with motion. Young men, clothed in nothing but a small strap, jumped off the mud walls, into the trees, and back down before jumping up again as if the earth was hot as coals. Their feet pounded with the tom-tom's beat and somehow did not trample the wrapped body that lay on the ground before them. They thrust their flaming millet stalks into the air and at each other, each one trying his best to withstand the heat, to subdue the flame.

Out of nowhere, a white chicken appeared in the center of the dancers and began to run wildly. Every man ran toward it, snatching frantically at the chicken with his torch-free hand while jabbing fire at his opponents with his other. What a race! As Louis had said, if one man gets the chicken, the others must grab it away, as this first man is trying to show he is stronger than everyone else. Finally, one man held onto the frightened fowl long enough to pull a knife and slit its throat. The white chicken had been killed, and the dead man's soul was released to the beyond. The dancers stopped, their feat accomplished.

John returned from Bamako with fantastic news. The birthing house project would be funded! Monique was elated, as were the dùgùtigi and the elders. The three of us had spent the day in Koutiala, ordering and pricing materials, eating lunch with Monique's family, and seeing Pascal briefly. Monique had headed back to the village early, having magically gotten the moped, and John and I were ready to return as well.

He put on his helmet, straddled the motorcycle, adjusted his new goat leather bag (purchased in Bamako, it was literally a hollowed-out goat, intended for use as a canteen in the desert but used as a carryall by volunteers) and kick-started the bike. I climbed on, my arms behind me to hold the back rack. We pulled out on to the main road and wove our way through town. Men in fatigues waved us through a roadblock. Two taxis and a bus were pulled over to the side. Travelers sat next to bundles of belongings while soldiers checked identification and poked through the vehicles.

John had said there was an eerie calm in Bamako. Expatriates did not go out at night. He'd heard a rumor that the Peace Corps bureau was reviewing evacuation plans—just in case. It was hard to believe that there was so much unrest in the capital. We hadn't seen any real sign of change around Koutiala, except for this increased military presence, and no change at all in the daily life of Nampossela.

Once through the center of town we turned left onto a dirt road that bisected a neighborhood before narrowing to a trail that spit us out onto the road to Nampossela. It was a shortcut that took a kilometer or so off our journey home. For a town road it was in bad shape, due in great part to the fact that it became a stream in the rains. It had dips and turns and waved left and right. I bounced and pitched on the back of John's motorcycle, gripping the rack more tightly as he weaved among the sandpits, roots, and rocks. He was so focused on our path that he didn't notice the two mobs until we were in the middle of them.

Movement to the right caught my eye. Emerging from behind a high wall was a group of fifty or so men carrying sticks and holding stones. I saw John look left. Another group was approaching fast from that side too.

The thin winding path did not allow a quick turn-around and the two groups would soon cut off our path forward. My breath tightened in my throat and I could feel John's arms shaking. John slammed on the brakes and put out a foot to keep us up. I jerked forward, hitting his back. Over the idling engine and through the insulated helmet I could hear a spray of angry words. I brought my head up as a young man burst through the front of the pack on the right and hurled a rock across the road. Missiles started flying in both directions, creating small explosions of dry dirt where they struck earth. A small group splintered off from the left and ran toward us, one man out in front, sticks raised high in the air and shouting. John checked behind us, then ahead, and started to gun the engine.

The leader, a man I didn't recognize, lowered his stick and put out his hands, stopping the advancing group.

"Fatumata? Bakary?" he shouted, squinting in the sun behind us. Though I did not recognize him, John and I both yelled, "Yes! Yes!" in reply.

He turned around, exchanging quick words with the men, who in turn yelled to the larger group behind them. The rock throwing ceased. Even the other mob settled down.

"Ah, Fatumata and Bakary *de don!*" he yelled to everyone, turning around for all to hear. "It is Fatumata and Bakary, let them through, it is Fatumata and Bakary of Nampossela."

The men stopped and let the ends of their sticks rest on the ground and the stones stay in their grips. A tense quiet filtered the settling dust.

"Merci."

John did not waste any time driving through the parted mobs. I glanced back as we picked up speed. Within seconds of our getaway, stones started flying and the fight was lost in clouds of dust. I shook with relief.

Though I didn't know what this fight was about, I knew there was the fever of revolution behind it. I felt an uncontrollable change coming. Like we had inadvertently fallen into something much bigger than ourselves. Something unpredictable.

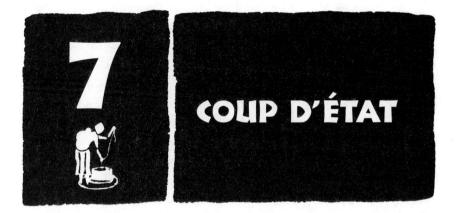

7

COUP D'ÉTAT

THE CROWD WAITING IN THE THIN SHADE OF THE CLINIC PORCH
GREETED ME, THOUGH PEOPLE WERE MORE SUBDUED THAN NORMAL.
They were listening to the static and Bambara coming from the small
dusty black box on Monique's desk. The radio was now Monique's
constant companion, as events in Bamako and elsewhere were happening
at a fast pace. Several students had been shot during a demonstration in
Bamako and others had been arrested and beaten. All schools were shut
down. In Koutiala, Pascal had given word that some prisoners had rioted
and attempted to escape. A few were shot and killed as they ran down the
main road.

Monique was examining an older woman whose hunched back was
toward the door. The woman's threadbare blue shirt lay crumpled next to
her on the examination slab. The patient turned to face me with slow
deliberateness. In both hands she gingerly cradled her left breast. It was
covered in small bumps and swollen to the size of an adult human head, so
different from the right one that fell limp against her belly. I stifled a gasp
as Monique came over to me.

"There are no signs of infection. It is cancer, I believe," Monique said in
French, her voice tense.

I didn't need to be a doctor to see that the woman needed a mastec-
tomy, at least.

I met the woman's hollow, beseeching gaze before looking away.

"What can you do?" I asked specifically, and then almost rhetorically,
"What do you do about cancer?"

Monique answered both questions with one word: nothing. Then, reaching for a grain of hope she said, "Perhaps if she went to Bamako . . ."

So she would die then.

Supporting the enlarged breast in the crook of her left arm, the woman used her right hand to pull on her shirt. She fumbled, and Monique stepped over to help, gently covering her shoulders. The woman nodded to Monique, then said good-bye and disappeared.

I sat down in the tippy metal chair. Basil was sitting in the far corner, his toddler attention held by an abandoned green flip-flop. He held it upright, then upside down, watching the broken toe strap droop. He chewed on it, sat on it, put it on his foot and tried to walk, then put it on his hand and tried to crawl. He saw me watching him, stopped, looked at his mom for reassurance, and returned to his play.

"Pascal is leaving," Monique said, looking up from her ledger. "To stop the war in Liberia. He is supposed to stay until there is peace. That could be a long time."

She took a deep, heaving breath and looked away.

"Oh, Monique. How dangerous is it?"

Danger. I could feel it creeping closer, waiting, like a scorpion wedged into a crevice of an old wall. Out of sight and poised to strike.

"Ah, I do not know." She kept looking down and shook her head. "He is part of a peace-keeping army to make sure the war does not spread across West Africa. I do not know what that means he will be doing. I know nothing about war."

I didn't either, but what I did know about Liberia told me it was a mess and I didn't want to imagine sweet, playful Pascal anywhere near it. Problems there had been brewing for decades. Founded in 1847 by ex-slaves returning from the U.S., Liberia's political history was unique in West Africa in that European powers had not mapped its borders. Despite this remarkable beginning, Liberia's successive totalitarian regimes had resulted in severe economic woes. As armed opposition groups fought to control the country, West African peacekeeping troops (or ECOMOS) were being called in to halt the spread of civil war.

"That's scary, Monique."

"Ah," she shrugged. "What can I do? I will listen to the radio. They have news every day about Malian soldiers in Liberia. They say how they are doing, and they list who was killed. In any case, he gave me this."

She held up her right hand, fingers pressed together. I looked at the three rings. There were the two I remembered, both silver-plated, both gently curving, one flat and the other with raised baroque swirls. The third ring was new. It was a hefty piece topped with a silver block, very masculine, that bore the initials "PK."

Pascal Konaté. I gulped.

"I'm not taking it off," Monique announced. "If someone asks me about the initials, I will tell him it is for my people, the people of Koutiala—*la Population de Koutiala.*"

For the next few hours, Monique and I did not sit down. Patient upon patient came through the door. I tended to the few I could serve, those needing pills or a simple wound dressing, rather than shots or diagnoses. By noon, there was still no sign that the work would taper off. The porch remained packed with bodies, moving their position with the shade. Basil had fallen asleep in a corner of the room, trimmings of cotton bandages he had found on the floor wadded into one hand and the flip-flop by his head.

A girl entered the clinic in a scented fog of perfume and hair gel, which told me she was not from Nampossela. She was well kept, her complet was crisp and new, her braids were free of stray hairs, and her black plastic high heels had all their sequins. The girl strolled to the examination slab, gave the ointment-stained surface a grimace before brushing it with her hand, and sat down. Her fine accoutrements and air of disdain could not hide the glassy look of fever in her eyes. She spoke to Monique in a hushed tone and held her abdomen as if it was causing her great pain. Then she glanced at me, covered part of her face in one hand, and lowered her voice to a whisper. Embarrassment needs no translator. I stepped outside.

After a few minutes, the girl walked past me, tucking tablets into her pagne. I went back in. Monique threw another syringe into the trash pile. Basil sat up, bleary-eyed. He began to holler, arms in the air, wanting to be picked up.

"Who is she?" I asked.

"She is the friend of the guy's girlfriend. They visit Nampossela together. I believe she is Adama's little friend."

Monique scowled, then walked over to Basil, who lay back down as she tried to pick him up.

"She is very sick, with a common disease, a sexual disease. She has discharge, pain, fever. I think it is called *gonorrhée* in French," Monique said as she walked away from Basil, who then sat up and began to cry again.

"Oh, this child! What do you want, Basil?"

She went back over and picked up the struggling Basil who was in the process of lying down again. She sat at the desk and reached into her bag on the floor, retrieving two brown bananas. She handed one to him, which he threw on the ground.

"You treated her?" I asked.

"Yes, though she did not have any money. I gave it to her on credit, as I have done before. She seems to have no trouble finding money for other things, though. But I told her if the man she is seeing does not get treated, then she will keep getting sick. How many times must she come to me for free treatment while the men do nothing? No shame. I tell you this; I will not give it to her free again. If *she* is going to keep infecting herself, then *he* must pay for it."

"I hate sitting and doing nothing," I said to John.

"Sucks." He replied while trimming the callused skin from around the deep dry cracks in his heel.

"Doesn't your mother hate that word?"

"Yep. There were only two things my brother and I had to promise never to do: never say 'suck,' and never ride a motorcycle."

A hefty chunk of skin flew from the end of his Swiss army knife scissors. Normally this would elicit a look of satisfaction, but John was lackluster. The enthusiasm and excitement that infused our myriad organizational meetings had dissipated, and so had the promised labor. Granted, the old roof and the failing concrete veneer had been chipped off, but that meant the new fragile building had to be put back together within the next three months. Before the rains. The workers had dwindled each consecutive day, until yesterday only Gawssou showed up. I looked around. I didn't see any workers coming.

Toward my right, set against a distant row of palms, a line of women snaked across the dry field. The line grew longer each day as village wells dried up. The women waited their turn at the only pump, a handle on top of a thin pipe descending a couple of hundred feet into an aquifer. Every once in a while a couple of women pointed and looked in our direction.

Most of them were excited about the project, but they weren't the ones who had to do the work. Building was a man's job.

We had been so careful to obtain permission from the decision makers in the village—the dùgùtigi and elder men. We listened and organized the effort according to their wishes, using local workers and resources. Monique had designed a low metal birthing table shaped like a chair with tiny legs to go on top of the large slab. It would have waterproof cushions, providing a soft place to squat and space enough for Monique's waiting hands. The local blacksmith was making the table as well as six new metal beds for resting, and a worktable for the delivery room. The project had all the markings of a Peace Corps volunteer's dream: village support and leadership, adequate funding, and the realizable result of improving women's and children's lives. I wanted so much for it all to happen; yet here John and I sat by the doorway, alone.

A blue dot far down the path slowly took form. Gawssou. His quick step and long, stork-like stride brought him to us in minutes. I tried not to stare at his skinny left thigh, exposed alongside a portion of white pocket through a huge rip in his pants.

"The villagers aren't coming," he said.

Gawssou was all business when there was work to be done.

"Why not?" John asked, stretched his legs and stood up.

"It started with the Konés. They refuse to come to work, as there is no millet beer. Everyone is now thinking about this and no one will come."

"Well," I said, "are we supposed to offer millet beer while they work?"

"Yes, and food, and a small amount of money," Gawssou said.

"The village is supplying the food and stipend. Remember?" I said, perturbed. It was hot and we had been over this so many times.

"Where is the food?" Gawssou said and looked around to prove his point. "I do not see any. It is not normal to have no food or drink."

"Sounds like yet another meeting to me!" John said with sarcastic enthusiasm, pulling me up and donning his wide brimmed straw hat. He was getting angry.

"There's something I want to talk to you about," I said to Monique, over her tinny radio perched on my windowsill. We sat across from each other in my small living room, Monique and Basil on the wood frame sofa, and I on the matching chair. She held the left side of her mouth gently in one hand. Her bad teeth were acting up today. Basil squirmed beside her, protesting her distraction.

"A women's group in Bamako that works on women's rights just sent me this on excision." I handed her a large envelope, which Basil tried to grab. Stepping over him, I took two aluminum spoons and a cooking pot off the counter and placed them on the floor. Monique set Basil down beside them and the banging commenced.

"You say there is a group in Bamako, speaking against this?" she asked in a loud voice.

"Yes, I ordered materials from four different organizations, and this is the only one that responded," I shouted.

"Can we . . ." her words and Basil's banging were both lost as a foraging flock of guinea fowl screeched and cackled just outside the window. "Can we read through them now?"

"Yes," I said and sat down next to her on the bench.

Basil gave up on the makeshift drum, crawled into the bedroom, pulled himself up by a high shelf, and tried to reach the books on it. He grunted in frustration.

Monique opened the materials: photocopied brochures, a staple-bound book, a small poster, and a cassette tape, all written in Bambara and French.

There were three levels of circumcision practiced across Africa. Circumcision, or *sunna*, entailed the removal of the hood of the clitoris and sometimes part of the clitoris itself; excision was the removal of the clitoris and all or part of the inner lips of the vagina; and infibulation meant the removal of the clitoris, inner lips, and all or part of the outer lips. Infibulation also entailed sewing the area back up and leaving a hole about the width of a matchstick. Though infibulation existed in Mali, it was more prevalent in East African nations, such as Sudan and Somalia. Excision was the form most common in Mali, universal really, with 96 percent of girls being cut. Although these practices were often justified on religious grounds, there is no mandate in any religious text, not in the Bible and not in the Koran.

A small number of excisions were performed in a hospital, under sterile conditions, but most girls were excised in dark huts with a razor blade, scissors, a knife, or a broken piece of glass. Very few of these tools were well cleaned. Some girls went into shock, some bled to death. Some lived only a few days longer before succumbing to blood poisoning or tetanus. Surviving in the short term did not guarantee that a girl's troubles were behind her. Recurrent tearing of the scar tissue during sex, permanent incontinence, and painful menstruation would many times become life-long companions. Bacterial infections were common, caused by the build-up of retained urine and menstrual fluid, and if an infection wormed its way into the womb, a woman was usually left infertile. Infertility also occurred in instances where a scarred vagina was particularly difficult for a man to enter and his repeated penetrations caused tears and damage to the perineum, urethra, and anus. The result was the opening up of a new hole, a "false vagina," a hole that did not lead to children.

Why did excision continue? Many believed that intact women were unable to control their sex drive, so it had to be controlled for them. Surprisingly, the older women were usually the practice's staunchest proponents. It was the only path to womanhood they knew. Without it, the future of the family was in jeopardy. Their daughters and granddaughters would be unsuitable marriage partners, and therefore unsuitable mothers, the one job each girl was born to do. The women who performed the excisions held one of the few revered positions that a woman could hold. On a personal level, doing away with excision meant a loss of power and income. They would not surrender that power without a fight.

"Ah, ah, ah," Monique said, when we finished. "Everything written here makes sense. It is right. The people in the cities, they are always thinking of new things, good things."

Then she held up the cassette and raised an eyebrow.

"It's in Bambara," I said. "It's meant to be played in women's groups, to begin a discussion."

"A good idea. Perhaps even my parents will listen to it. My youngest sister has yet to be cut." Monique clicked her tongue in the back of her throat.

"There are women's movements in other African countries, like Senegal. They are speaking out against the practice." I added, "They, too, say that girls should remain intact, that there are ways of keeping the ritual of becoming a woman without the cutting."

A loud bang came from the bedroom as Basil, having given up on the bookshelf, raised the lid on John's metal trunk. He began to empty out all the papers and folders. I went over and put them all back. He waited for me to leave and took them out. He was exhaustingly repetitious, but at least he was occupied.

"So, what they call the most pleasurable spots are what is removed?" Monique asked.

"Yes, where the nerve endings are." I sat back down beside her and pointed at the diagram in the book. "There."

"Women, who have these parts," her eyes flamed in her face, "can feel pleasure as great as a man's?"

"Yes, as far as I know," I nodded.

"Ba, ba, ba," Monique said in surprise, tapping her closed fist against her lips in disbelief. "You, you have had this kind of pleasure?"

"With some men, yes, and with some, no. Men still have it easier, with all the pleasure parts hanging on the outside. For the woman, it depends on whom she is with. If the man tries to please her or not."

She clicked.

"Yes, this is true. There are men who are rough and men who are gentle."

She played with her ring, the *PK* swirling in and out of sight as she twisted it round.

"Some men just don't know what they're doing!" I laughed. "But, to be fair, it's not like women always know what to ask for. Even in my country, where we have our female parts intact, we are not taught how to talk about sex and pleasure."

"And for your first time? Did you have pain then?"

"Yes, there was some blood. There's still a small membrane that breaks, even when you haven't been excised."

Monique nodded, cupping her face in both of her hands, and leaned over, elbows on spread knees.

"What about you, Monique?"

"My first time?" she dropped her hands and her face scrunched up in thought. "It hurt, a lot. An older boy I had seen before took me into his hut; it was very dark. I tried to get away, but he held me down, on the mat, and then, that was it."

"He forced you?"

"Yes," she shrugged. "It was painful and then it was over."

"Oh . . ." I said, my face suddenly warm.

"It's okay," she said, "it was a long time ago. You have not heard of this either?"

"I have."

"What's wrong?"

A memory, rarely spoken, escaped and flowed into my mouth, swelled my tongue and choked my speech, "Something like that happened to me, too. Being forced, by a boy."

"Ah, Fatumata, it was this way for me, and for other of my friends," Monique said, looking at me with a mixture of concern and confusion. She paused for a moment, watching me, moving slightly closer. "It is normal. It happens."

Her words made me feel less alone, safer. Yet I couldn't imagine that Monique, or anyone else, could think being forced to have sex was normal. But she hadn't called it rape, or anything violent. I had read about women and internalized repression, was this a sign of it? Rape, or forced sex, or whatever term one wanted to apply, was a reality faced by women all over the world, but Monique didn't seem to have baggage, no perception that she had somehow been violated, no shame or self-reproaching. That, I knew, was a great thing.

John and I walked toward the family compound for lunch after another exhausting morning at the birthing house. The day had started out with a meeting at the clinic in which the dùgùtigi, giant hands folded humbly in his lap, had told us of Nampossela's debt to CMDT. To help pay off this debt, CMDT had kept 2 million CFA of the village's cotton money (about $4,000) and hence the village was broke. This was why our communal work parties weren't well attended. Not only were people angry at reduced profits, but they also knew the village didn't have the means to provide food and beer for the birthing house construction. Nampossela could not keep its end of the bargain. According to the terms of our grant from USAID, if the village backed out, the funds were to be returned. The project died where it was.

The failing project occupied our thoughts as we walked. As the heat surged from the high sun, all seemed baked still; nothing moved along the path but our stunted shadows. An old man sat, slowly weaving cotton on a rough, handmade loom under the thick protection of a mango tree.

The strips, used to make mudcloth, were long enough to swathe the neck of a giraffe.

"Fatumata, Bakary," came the dùgùtigi's voice from afar and on high. Startled, John and I stopped and looked across the roofs of the huts to either side of us. "Up here."

We looked ahead along the path to where it opened up onto another communal area and saw the rustling of dusty greens high in the branches of an ancient néré. As we approached, we heard the clacking of seedpods and could just see him, balanced near the tapered end of a thick branch. One hand gripped a higher branch while the other reached for the long, brown envelopes of precious black seeds needed to make the spice sunbala.

"How's the collecting?" I asked. "Mawa has put you to good use."

"Yes, she has," he said, squatting on the branch and peering down at us. "I have news. On the radio, they said there has been a coup d'état. President Moussa Traoré has been arrested by the military. They captured Traoré's wife at the airport as she was trying to get away. They captured her in a plane full of gold."

The dùgùtigi took one hard breath, and then shook his head. "Hundreds of people were killed in the fight; many buildings burned. It is said that Bamako overflows with smoke and blood."

I looked at John and watched as fear shadowed his face.

"Oh my God," I said, and leaned into him.

The dùgùtigi saw my reaction and switched his tone.

"Fatumata and Bakary, you will be safe here. You will not have problems."

"We know," John said, gently leading me by the hand to go, "but we have to find out what the Peace Corps needs us to do."

Peace Corps plans called for us to listen to the news on the shortwave in the event of the government's fall. If the news said that volunteers in Mali were to proceed to "A," then we were to evacuate, mounted atop our motorcycles, and head to the border with Burkina Faso, two hours east. No formal good-byes, no packing up, just leaving with our passports, knapsacks, and unfinished dreams. Monique's last image of us would be our yellow helmets, vanishing into the distance like planets released from their orbits.

"I want to find Monique," I said.

We walked at a brisk pace toward the outskirts of town, leaving the dùgùtigi to his picking, all thoughts of the birthing house project swept out by the rush of adrenaline. John headed to our house and our radio while I ran to the clinic, almost plowing into the people waiting on the porch. I pushed through them and entered.

"Monique."

She was bending down, her head lost in the medicine cabinets, bottles in each hand. Startled, she turned around and stood up.

"Monique, did you hear the news that there has been a coup d'état today? The dùgùtigi just told me."

Four of five women from the porch gathered in the doorway and asked me what was wrong. Before I could respond, Monique explained in Bambara what I had asked.

"Ohhhhh," they responded and went back outside.

"Yes, I heard it on the radio," Monique said, laying the bottles on the table and selecting a vial. "The students, they finally got what they wanted. At least this will mean an end to the riots."

"And hopefully an end to military rule," I said. She eyed me as if waiting to hear what else I had to say.

"You look afraid, Fatumata, but you should not be."

She started filling a syringe with the clear fluid of the antibiotic vial, *Gentamicin.*

"But Monique, if the Peace Corps feels volunteers are in danger, if there is more violence in the cities, we may be evacuated."

"Evacuated? This is true?"

I nodded. She dropped the syringe.

"Bakary went just now to listen to the radio. They have a signal they'll give if we have to leave for Burkina Faso."

Monique picked up the syringe and threw it in the corner where the day's waste had accumulated and would soon be taken and dumped outside in the ever-growing pile. She looked down at her hands and said, "The Peace Corps should know that nothing will happen here in the village. Even if the government changes in Bamako, nothing will change in Nampossela. They should know that. Fatumata, this is serious." Her broad shoulders sank into her chest. "What will I do here without you? I will be all alone."

During the next weeks, all borders remained closed and all government functions disrupted. John and I waited to hear what the new leader, General Amadou Touré, would actually do. Yes, he was military, but he promised to oversee real elections. No evacuation had been issued yet, just the same messages to stay put and keep listening.

I went to the clinic with the birthing house project proposal in hand, trying desperately to concentrate on it. I walked with a heavy foot, partly from sadness at the prospect of being whisked away, partly from the desire to ground myself, as if the pounding of my feet could signal my firm resolve to stay. As soon as I arrived, Monique asked for news.

"We're just supposed to stay put."

"Voilà. Good advice. Is this not what I told you? Eh?" Monique said. Her mocking superiority didn't hide her relief or soften her drawn, tired face. "I'm glad for that, as it seems all my friends are leaving me. It is Korotun who now has left."

"She's left?"

"She has returned to the village of her birth. She asked me to tell you and to say good-bye. She left last night. Dramane wasn't home." She paused, her eyes soft and apologetic. "She wanted to say good-bye to you, but I think she was right to leave quickly. Things were only getting worse between them."

"Will her family take her back?"

"That, I do not know. But I hope that when she explains what has been happening, they will see she had no other choice. She has only one child, she should be able to find another husband one day."

"What about Ami? Dramane certainly can't take care of her."

"She took Ami. Dramane claims a child as his own only if it is a boy," Monique said. She walked past me and hailed the next patient, a young woman from the Koulibaly quarter, here for a shot of vitamin A. The baby on her back, evidently afraid he would be the one to be poked and prodded, began a high, moaning wail as Monique ignored the crying and eased the needle under the mother's skin.

An older man from the Kelema family entered. Severe headaches, he stated. Monique asked a few questions, discerned that it was not malaria, and then nodded toward the aspirin drawer. I gave him two individually wrapped pills in exchange for a few palm-warmed coins. Monique reminded him to drink more water, make sure it was clean, and avoid dòlo. She sat down at her desk. As there were no more patients, I sat down in the chair by the door and flipped to the budget page of the birthing-house materials.

"Monique, let's talk about what we can trim from the project." Gut or gouge would have been more appropriate terms, but I wanted to work on it. Planning it, even if it meant scaling way back, meant that I had a future here. "Maybe we can still save it."

"This is difficult," she answered me, elbows on her desk.

"Yes, but we have to decide. Bakary and I think that we can't cut back on the birthing house itself. The recementing of the walls, and the shoring up of the eroded corners, roof, and beams have got to be done."

"We don't have to repair the nyegens," she said.

"No, we don't," I said, "but that'll mean the women must stop using them soon. The floors are caving in."

"They can still bathe in one corner of the left one and when that goes, they can bathe at home. But I do want to complete at least one well," she said.

"So, we can leave off the other well . . ."

"I want to do the birthing table."

"Yes, that's important. And, the work has already begun on it," I said, going over the items again. "The remaining high-cost items are the six new beds, including their mattresses, sheets, and pillows; three chairs; and your medicine and supply storage trunk."

"Perhaps we can do . . ." Monique said. "We can do two beds, not six. No chairs or storage trunk."

I did the calculations.

"Still not enough. Let's see, if I take out all the beds . . . that's it. If we don't purchase any of the supplies for the resting rooms, we can still do one well, repair the building, and do the birthing table."

"Then that's what we must do," Monique said and nodded.

Later that day, the dùgùtigi and twelve elderly village men with kola nut stained teeth listened as John and I explained how much the pared down version of the birthing house would cost. After much discussion, they agreed and said they could definitely come up with the reduced amount of food and drink. On the walk back to our house, the dùgùtigi admitted to us that the village would come up with their share by forcing those villagers most in debt to the village to "donate" chicken, sheep, or millet beer for the workers. An unsavory situation indeed.

John and I lay in bed that night, uncomfortably hot, bodies restless, minds whirring. Then we heard a ping on the roof. Another ping and more until the tin hummed: a mango rain. For an hour, everything came alive, and we breathed the scent of the trees and land again, inhaling the scent of hope and a new start, and finally fell asleep.

Blanche and Elise, who were handspinning raw cotton into thread, mesmerized me. They sat next to each other on the ground, legs straight out in front. On a scrap of leather, they twirled a sharpened stick like a top with one hand, thumb and forefinger guiding the string onto the stick, while the other hand held the fluff of cotton taut. The large looms to make cloth were a man's domain—the thread to hold the cloth together, a woman's. Mother and daughter worked in flawless, even rhythm.

Karamogo sat beside his mom, dry skin pulled over his bloated belly, staring at the small bowl of food Monique had placed in front of him. Elise made no move to help him eat. François was bathing in the nyegen. John was sitting with Louis, sharing a gourd of tangy millet beer, and listening to the old one's war stories. Louis reclined in his chair, his heels in and craggy toes splayed out. His arms gesticulated the marches, guns, and explosions he encountered while fighting. John leaned forward in his chair, partly from interest, but partly, I knew, in an attempt to understand Louis' husky slurred words.

"You didn't eat much chicken tonight Fatumata," Monique said with a wink as she cleared away the bowl. Louis had killed two scrawny fowl in our honor. Though I'd been eating with the family for a year and a half, he still couldn't grasp the fact that I didn't eat meat.

"Nope, yet again, I must leave the delicious bits for someone else," I said.

"Are many Americans vegetarians like you?" Monique asked.

"No," I chuckled, "most Americans are definitely *not* vegetarians. They eat meat at almost every meal. As for me, I never liked meat, even as a little girl. I never saw a reason for killing animals, since I could survive without eating them. But since living here in Nampossela, where people don't always have enough to eat, I can see a reason for killing to eat. Before living here, I had always valued animals almost as much as humans."

"This is true?" Monique asked, eyes wide with disbelief.

"Yes," I said, "In the U.S., we're very attached to our pets, mostly cats and dogs. They live inside with us, sleep in our beds, go to the doctor. Stores even sell special food, just for them. I guess you could say that for some people, their dog or cat is their closest friend."

She shook her head, turned, and carried the bowls into the cooking hut. How could I possibly explain how we related to our pets in the U.S.? It did seem bizarre, now that I thought about it, and such a luxury to care for animals as humans. I still had no desire to eat meat, but I did feel differently about animals' deaths. Recently in a neighboring village, I had seen the *Nyakajugu* (ugly fétiche) ceremony, so named for the grotesque mass of blackened horns and roots of this fétiche, covered in decades of blood. I had seen sheep, goats, and, yes, dogs sacrificed and knew what the "watering" of the fétiche meant. The féticheur and his supplicants held the bleating or growling animal, stretched taut its neck and quickly cut, letting the blood flow over the sacred object. How could I possibly explain to my friends at home that I wasn't horrified? Even when offered a skinned, boiled, and seasoned piece of Fido? Somehow the sacred, communal ritual brought honor and reason to the deaths, something no one had done for the cows that made up the fast-food burgers back home. If I was ever to eat meat, I'd rather it be here.

John came over and sat next to me, interrupting my carnivorous musings.

"In no way," he said with a yawn, "does dòlo help me understand Louis."

"Has it helped you come up with a solution for the birthing house?"

"Nope. At least nothing grand. I just know that doing something is better than nothing."

"And coercive or not," I said, "I do love the idea of men donating their meat, beer, and labor for the betterment of women and children."

We sat in thought. Then I had an idea.

"What if we got some private donations?"

"You mean, ask other cash-strapped Peace Corps volunteers for money?"

"No, ask our families back home, and friends. My parents have offered to help us, if we need it. I bet their church could pull together some funds. They're itching to do mission work."

"We'll have to get the money over here fast, which is no easy feat," he said. "A wire transfer to the Bank of Africa, somehow . . . but it's possible. We'll need to look at the figures again, so we know exactly how much money we need and make a list of who to contact and how. Maybe people could buy a specific item—'your twenty dollars will buy a beautiful, polyester-covered mattress, or two delicious sheep.'"

"What are you two talking about?" Monique asked, coming out of the cooking hut with two pots in each hand, and noticing our excitement. John explained our plans as she dumped the leftover couscous into the smaller of the two containers.

"Hey!" she said, and then put down the pots and clapped her hands on her thighs. "That would be so good."

I got up to help clean, grabbed a stubby broom, and swept the bits of food, stray millet stalks, and wind-blown dirt into a pile. François walked out of the nyegen, plopped his empty bucket down by the cooking hut, the metal handle falling to one side with a bang, and sat down by his father. He picked up his radio and turned it on, loud.

"Another good project has come up as well," Monique said, glancing at François as music and static filled the air.

I stopped sweeping as she came closer.

"I met with the Koutiala director of World Vision, the one who works on health projects here. She said that if we teach all the women in the village how to make keneya ji—the oral rehydration drink—World Vision will supply us with free birth control pills. They will come out to Nampossela and test the women on this. If all the women pass and if at least fifteen women are interested in birth control, we can store the pills here, in Nampossela."

I swept with renewed vigor.

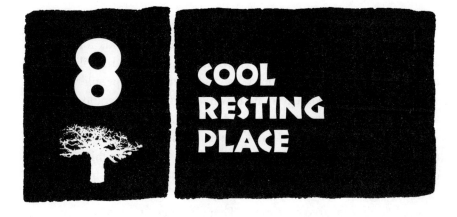

8 COOL RESTING PLACE

THE BIRTHING HOUSE LOOKED LESS LIKE A RENOVATION THAN AN ERUPTED VOLCANO. The top was gone, clouds of red dust billowed out the empty window and door frames. As if they had exploded from within, the old beds, stained foam mattresses, and plastic sheets lay strewn about the grounds. The discarded tin roof and termite-attacked beams had been scavenged. Only rubble piles of veneer chips and broken bricks were left behind. Two Koulibaly men scraped away at the northwest corner like dentists cleaning out a large cavity. Gawssou was shoveling and pushing scattered debris into piles, and John was carefully checking newly molded bricks to see if they were dry. Even the dùgùtigi was wandering around the work site, lending a hand. As usual, no Konés had shown.

John jumped back from a brick. The workers laughed.

"I hate scorpions," he said in English and looked at me. "That's the fourteenth one I've found this morning. I'm doing something else for awhile."

His body shivered as he picked up a hoe to help.

I found a broom and joined three other Dembele women who were cleaning out the rooms. We spent most of the morning bent over, sweeping and hauling out heavy debris. We wrapped old pagnes around the end of long sticks, dipped them in buckets of water, and splashed them around the floor. The first pass left a thick film of mud, but subsequent mops eliminated most of the dirt. By noon, I was spent.

So far, each quartier had made bricks and provided donkey carts of sand and gravel for the concrete. That had been relatively easy. The trips across the village did not take too much time, but finding people to lend their carts for longer trips, like to Koutiala for bags of cement and roofing, was another matter. It was time to prepare the fields for planting. Hands were needed for clearing, turning the earth, and fertilizing, and donkey carts were the primary transportation for people and cow manure. As a result, there were no new materials and we would soon be at a point where no amount of food or drink would lure workers.

But it was good to be back in the messiness of it all with the threat of evacuation over. The killing had stopped with the coup, while a few student protests lingered. The country was in a state of shock and tranquility. Posters, stickers, and clothes picturing the now deposed Moussa Traoré had disappeared over night. There had been fears of retaliation, of Moussa's supporters rallying together for a counterattack, but as the weeks passed and the entire military expressed its allegiance to the new leadership, people dared think the impossible: democracy. Other Malians remained fearful, but not of the military. They feared Allah's wrath. Hundreds had died at the hands of their countrymen. How might Mali be punished?

The coup had made contacting friends and family back home even more difficult than usual. The country's infrastructure was still being patched back together. Mail, phones, and wires were down. John and I decided to act on faith. We figured that we would get the money from the U.S. at some later date, and bought supplies on credit. We just hoped that nobody would collect early.

Through the scratchy sound of my sweeping, I heard the scrape and chink of shoveling stop. I stood up, broom in hand, and arched my back. Elise's voice announced the arrival of lunch. Gawssou, the dùgùtigi, and John walked toward the entrance and through the streaks of sunlight. I followed them outside, brushing grime off my dress. In the brilliance of day, clumps of children had collected to watch the big project like they would gather at a construction site in the U.S., although I thought my broom a poor substitute for a bulldozer.

We all walked toward the well to wash off. A donkey sniffed the ground, evidently looking for water too. The girls filling buckets shooed him off. Next to me, the Koulibaly men, who had also stopped their work, began to grumble.

"If the Konés were here, this work would be finished."

"They had better come tomorrow."

One man took his plastic teapot, his salidaga, just filled by one of the girls, leaned over, and washed the grit from his face. He shook his hands dry.

The donkey let loose a horrendous bray that drowned out every other noise, seesawing until it petered out between vibrating hairy lips. I may have grown up in farm country, but before coming to Mali I had no idea how loud a donkey could bray, especially the males. They would make a racket and, more often than not, follow it up with an obscenely huge erection. A second deafening bray. A growing member. One of the Koulibalys picked up a small stone and hurled it at the beast to drive it away. It harmlessly bounced off the belly. He tossed another and hit the same spot. The animal only seemed to get more aroused and, to add insult, turned his hindquarters in our direction. He hee-hawed at us from over his shoulder and undulated his hips. We were being mocked. No wonder a donkey is called an ass. Another small stone finally sent the beast on his way.

Chuckling, I looked at John. From his devilish grin, I knew that we were thinking of a similar incident in his former village of Sanso. If John hadn't sworn he had seen it himself, I never would have believed it.

The tale began with workers driving off a feisty donkey, but one projectile found a most surprising target. It stuck in the beast's anus. The donkey gulped in mid-bray. He groaned, flexed, and urgently swished his tail. He turned his head this way and that and pushed his hips in every direction. John and the workers fell to the ground and slapped themselves as they exploded in laughter. The more the donkey worked at dislodging the stone, the more the men responded. They had trouble breathing. Some coughed. The donkey stared straight at the ground, and with a look of powerful concentration, it pushed out its rear. The rock quivered, reluctant to abandon its warm home, and dropped. With two snorts the donkey trotted off. One boy ran over to where the moistened missile lay in the dirt, but John shook his head and told him to leave it alone. For months, John heard the men recounting the story to one another, picking up stones as props and mimicking the donkey's actions.

We walked away from the well and toward a giant, fortress-like baobab tree. Birds squawked and darted about, retreating now and then into the leaves. Elise and two young girls had arranged the bowls of rice, sauce, and beer in the tree's mottled shade. As we approached, the dùgùtigi's smile turned to a thin line as he looked out to the fields and scrubby brush in the distance.

"The fields are dry, Bakary," he said.

"Very dry," John agreed.

"If the rains do not come this year," the dùgùtigi continued, "we will all go back to America with you when you leave."

I smiled at the thought, but looked up to see that he did not.

It was early May, the preamble to the rainy season and the most tense month. Healthy rains mean life and poor rains mean death, and there was no telling which a year would bring. Severe droughts in the seventies and early eighties were burned into the memories of many villagers. I wondered if it was always this way, when existence depended on circumstances beyond human control. Not that a measure of control was not tried. Animals were sacrificed, prayers were made, but everyone knew that in the end it was not blood and words that let the village live, it was the will of God. Little wonder everybody was so anxious.

The men took their places. The dùgùtigi, Gawssou, and John waited for me, their wet hands dangling. The women were sitting around another bowl of rice, also waiting. I didn't feel like eating hot, sticky rice on a hot, sticky afternoon.

"Please, go ahead and eat," I said.

They attacked the food before I finished my sentence. I walked over to Elise and told her to please eat with the other women, and make sure that Karamogo got some soft pieces of chicken. I looked at her toddler, hanging loosely off her back like a bundle of sticks. No amount of bra-promising, baby-weighing, or food-demonstrating had stopped her habit of ignoring him. Elise sat down at the bowl and put Karamogo in her lap. She put a small piece of chicken up to Karamogo's tiny cracked lips. He sat there, at first not responding. Then I watched him struggle to swallow, as if his body had forgotten or never learned how.

I decided to walk to the clinic and let Monique know how the work on the birthing house was coming along. When I arrived, the door was open, but no women were there. Monique sat, eyes closed, her head resting on one outstretched arm along the desk, as she listened to soft music coming from the radio on the window sill. A Bic pen moved back and forth in her left hand, creating a deep blue groove in the top of the desk. Basil slept on a pagne. Flies crawled over his food-stained yellow t-shirt and diaper-free derrière. She looked up as I entered.

"Hi Monique, where is everyone? Didn't you have keneya ji and baby food demonstrations today?"

"Yes, but they have all gone to the fields," she said through a yawn.

Monique had been giving crash courses throughout the quartiers all week. The local branch of World Vision would come to Nampossela within the month to assess the women's knowledge of diarrhea and oral rehydration. I wasn't sure this was the most effective way to improve kids' health, but it was the easiest way for Monique to demonstrate what the women had learned. And if we could prove we were teaching women how to care for their children, we could stock free birth control pills. Yes, there were good reasons to have large families: more hands to help with myriad duties that life demanded and more help for parents in their elder years. But it also meant more mouths to feed and, with each child after the fourth or fifth, greater danger in childbirth for the mother. If women wanted to control how many children they had, reliable birth control was a good first step.

"Fatumata, I have lost the ring."

"What?"

"*His* ring."

She glanced at me, then pointed to her hand. The large silver square was gone.

"Where do you think you lost it?"

"I don't know. But it is not a good sign. It is not a good sign at all."

She sighed and shook her head. "I have received no letters from him in weeks."

"But the mail hasn't been dependable since the coup. And couldn't it just mean that he's far away, without a way to get one to you?"

"That is what I told myself, until losing the ring. Something is not right. It is a sign," she said as she tilted her head toward the radio, wanting to catch every word through the sputters and crackles. "I keep listening and every minute I pray that I will continue to hear nothing."

It was time to see Mariko again. Surely, if we could make progress on a complex village project like the birthing house, we could get Monique her salary. Or so I thought. We passed the ever-growing heap of medical waste, not far from the clinic entrance. Two children played in its bloodied bandages, fluid-stained cotton wipes, and fluttery plastic pill wrappers. Each child clutched a used syringe.

"Hey!" John yelled from under his wide-brimmed straw hat. "Get out of there!"

The two young boys dropped the goods, ran behind the guesthouse and peeked back around the corner, waiting for a chance to return.

"We should actually do something about that," John said.

Monique's increase in patients meant an increase in trash. Inorganic refuse was an unfortunate and, in this case, dangerous by-product. She was being more careful about what she threw where, but options were limited without curbside pickup.

"We've got to dig a waste pit for all this." John said and walked closer to the pile.

"Like a nyegen?"

"Yes, a deep one. I'll ask Daouda, the well-digger. I can make the concrete cover and leave a small hole in it so Monique can empty the trash, but nothing else can get down there, and nothing can be pulled out. Should last for a few years."

"Another project. Just add it to the list," I said.

We picked through the top of the trash, taking out the more dangerous items and disposed of them in our own nyegen. Then we got on our motorcycle and headed west, to the hospital. I thought the presence of a man would lend more weight to Monique's cause.

But I was wrong. Mariko, sitting and rustling forms, gave the same pleasantries and promises to John as he had to me. It was almost maddening. There was some good news; getting Henri Traoré trained as an official health agent was not difficult at all. It was a matter of funds to pay for training and then a matter of registering him. Monique had said the training was 150,000 CFA. Three hundred dollars. If John and I each saved part of our monthly stipend, and cashed in some of our emergency traveler's checks, we could do it.

Gawssou was at our door, gently rapping in the early morning light, before John and I had taken our bucket baths, before we had even lit the fire on the gas stove.

"Bakary, Fatumata," Gawssou said, glancing up from his feet only to look directly at ours. "You must come see my daughter. I think she is very sick."

"What's happening?" John asked.

"She has diarrhea, and she is very hot."

"When did it start?"

"Ah," he made an empty shrug, still looking down. "A long time ago. But it is becoming worse."

I joined John on the porch, sending a lizard, looking to bask in the first rays of daylight, scuttling away. "How old is she?"

"Salimata is two, maybe three years. She is my youngest daughter."

My mind ran through the people we had seen in the clinic over the past few days and I didn't remember seeing his second wife Fatim or his child.

John looked at the almost hidden face of Gawssou then looked at me, "I'll go with him now."

"The World Vision people are coming out this morning. They'll be here within an hour," I said. "Maybe Monique or I can leave early."

John and I ducked inside to collect the plastic bags filled with salt and sugar for the rehydration drink.

"Why did Gawssou come to us and not Monique?" John asked quietly in English.

"I don't know. Maybe he went to Monique too."

"Maybe. He's never asked us for anything before."

Within minutes Gawssou and John left. I took a quick bucket bath and by the time I was done, the clinic was open and a few women had gathered across the field, under the shade of a large hangar. Others began to arrive from all directions, all on foot.

Monique had on a new pagne, green, yellow, and black horizontal striped with shiny golden threads woven throughout it, and a clean white shirt. She sparkled, ready to receive our guests. I told her of Gawssou's early visit to our home. He had mentioned nothing to her.

"His wife has not brought Sali into the clinic," Monique said. "But she is quiet like Gawssou. I am worried that for him to ask this of you means it could be very serious. We must go to her as soon as this is over."

We closed the clinic, gathered the buckets of pump water Monique had fetched, and took them, a cream-colored bowl, a large liter-size plastic cup, a spoon, and the sugar and salt, and joined the growing crowd. Like Monique, they were all dressed in their best: crisp, brightly colored pagnes with embroidered collars and matching headscarves. Receiving guests seemed to bring out the best in everyone, even if they were exhausted with worry over the lack of rain. Mawa and the twins arrived, one boy strapped to his mother's hefty frame while a small girl wrestled under the weight of the other. There was Oumou, baby girl on her back; there was Kadjatou and little William. Everyone was taking a seat, like flocks of birds settling on the shore.

Soon a massive white four-wheel-drive Toyota Landcruiser thundered into town. The driver, a thin man with a pack of Dunhills in his chest pocket ambled out and opened the doors for two large, stylishly attired women. They were both in fancy *boubous* (long, shiny waxed gowns made of the finest woven cotton), which flowed over their plentiful frames, just touching the tops of their faux leather high heels. Their braided hair was streaked with golden strands, and coiled around their heads in tight beehives. The women introduced themselves to me and greeted Monique. Mme. Keita and Mme. Bagayogo were from away—their names were Bambara, not Minianka, and their accents were those most often heard on the streets of Bamako. They wiggled into their chairs, pulled out some graph paper and pens, and the test began.

Mme. Keita cleared her throat and posed her questions. "When do you give keneya ji to a child?" "What are the causes of diarrhea?" "Why is rehydration important?" Mme. Bagayogo made notes between glances into the audience and asked women to come forward and demonstrate how to make the rehydration concoction.

Monique stood at Mme. Keita's side, first encouraging women to speak, then nodding when they responded correctly. Monique guided and led as needed, taking the threads of the women's knowledge and joining them together, creating a fabric of wisdom. As I observed the trio, I realized how much Monique fit in. Though she lacked their education, their driver and car, their imported fancy cloth, and her wide feet would never conform to heels, she too stood elegantly and confidently in front of the crowd. Her role as a leader was natural.

After a couple of hours, the Madames were impressed. They tossed communal good-byes to the women who then quickly dispersed to their waiting chores. Monique and I walked the ladies to their vehicle, woke the driver, and watched their gleaming Toyota drive off.

"So, we did well on the test, right?" I asked, relieved that it was over, yet doubtful of its significance. What they could not test was the future. Would the villagers know when to make it? Would they use clean water? Would they have money to buy the sugar?

"We did very well," Monique said. "I think they were pleased."

"What about the birth control, then?

"I don't think they can deny us."

I smiled. Yet there was no time to relish this potential success, as Monique and I were due at Gawssou's home on the other side of Nampossela.

"Aw ni ce," we called as we entered the empty compound. Four children appeared from around the corner of a granary. Their piercing eyes and gentle grins said they were Gawssou's. They stood, huddled together, staring at me.

"Aw ni ce," came Gawssou's voice from within the small straw-roofed hut facing me.

"We're in here," said John.

I squinted into the darkness as Monique and I stepped over the dirt threshold of the doorway and into the one-room structure. The heat and breath of people enveloped us. Slowly I made out three adult figures, sitting on the ground, and three moving bodies in a corner, children. The four children outside followed and stood, silhouetted in the entrance, blocking the light. I slowed my breathing.

"I ni ce," came a soft voice. It must be Fatim, Gawssou's wife.

My eyes adjusted. A thin stream of white light came in through the tiny window. Rolled straw mats were piled in one corner, and gourds hung from the ceiling on ropes, filled with a jumble of objects I could not make out. The earth floor was as smooth as marble. Fatim sat with outstretched legs under her large pregnant belly. Beside her was Sali, staring to one side and arms up by her head.

I could feel Monique take in the room, the quiet, the sense of suffering.

"She is very sick," Gawssou said. He turned a weak flashlight on Sali's face. Two glass eyes sat in sunken flesh. Her hair was thin, her belly swollen, and her limbs wasted. No doubt about it, she had *kwashiorkor,* a type of malnutrition caused by a severe lack of protein. Monique knelt down, gently turned the child's head, looked in her eyes, and felt her arms and legs.

"We made keneya ji," John said, "but she won't drink it. She won't even take a sip. And she won't eat either." His voice cracked as he spoke. I couldn't make out John's face, just the shape of his head. I longed to reach for his hand. It dawned on me then, why they had come to John and me first. They came in hope of magic, white people's magic. Some part of them knew it had come to that.

Monique took out her stethoscope and listened to Sali's heart and her breathing, then gently, slowly rewrapped her.

"You must take her to Koutiala," Monique said, never shifting her gaze from the child, "to the hospital. There they can give her shots to stimulate her appetite, shots of vitamins. But, Gawssou, you must know that these shots are expensive. They are 2,500 CFA."

Five times what a laborer is paid in a day.

"There is no money," said Gawssou. He rose to his feet, clapped his hands together and then moved them apart, allowing them to hang empty in the air, as if beckoning a miracle from the sky.

John and I looked at each other. We were thinking the same thing—we had the money. It felt awkward, this power we had because of money. White people's magic. The power to save or not save. And it wasn't so much the power itself as how, in times like this, it disrupted the more give-and-take, egalitarian relationship we so cherished with our friends. But the choice was clear.

"No, Gawssou, we'll get you the money," John said, then stood up and walked out the doorway at a clip.

"If my moped is here, you can take it, Gawssou," Monique said, and also walked out. Gawssou followed. Fatim got up to put on new clothes for the journey.

It wasn't until later in the afternoon the next day that Gawssou told us. I'd wondered if we should go to his house and inquire, but then thought better of it. Monique said he would come to our house when he had news.

He walked through the gate door, rapping lightly. The heat had taken its toll, and John and I were napping on mats on the porch. We quickly arose.

"Gawssou," John said, standing up and searching his face. "How are you?"

"I looked for you at the well by the birthing house, but everyone was already gone." His eyes were almost lost under the wide lip of his blue cap.

"I came to tell you that I have returned from Koutiala. I thank you for paying for the medicine for my daughter, to bring her back to health. But God did not want it. My daughter, she died yesterday. Just before she died, she asked for water, and she received it from Fatim and from me."

Monique had explained that the dying often ask for a drink, and taking one guarantees against eternal thirst.

"I buried her last night in Nampossela. May the earth be light upon her."

"Gawssou," John sighed, "Gawssou . . ." His Bambara failed him as he reached out to touch his friend. "I'm so sorry," he said, in English, forgetting.

Gawssou kept his hand in John's and nodded. Then he walked to our salidaga and poured a steady stream of water over his hands and face. He walked back to us and sat down. We sat in silence. His hands turned from glistening black to dry brown as the sky took up its drops.

I got off the foam mattress without a sound. John was still sleeping, but I'd been watching a lizard on the wall for what seemed like hours. I thought about Gawssou and Fatim, and I thought about the rains. If they came too soon, they could destroy the birthing house, too late, and the crops and in turn my friends would suffer. I grabbed my pagne that lay crumpled on the floor, and began to wrap it around myself when something fell down my leg, making a hollow clack as it hit the floor. Beside my left foot was a seven-inch long, jet-black scorpion. It stretched one bent limb, opened its claws, and curled its tail.

My shriek sent John careening from the covers.

Unable to speak, I pointed at the creature that was now advancing toward me. John ran into the front room, and grabbed a sharp dàba. As he got behind it, the giant arachnid started to turn to face him. John brought down the blade of the hoe and cut off the tail. Scissoring claws cut the air. He turned the dàba around, letting the creature grasp the handle, then brought the dangling scorpion beyond the compound's wall where he smashed it. I gathered the courage to scoop up the tail's end between two forks and dump it beside the flattened corpse. Within minutes, foraging ants found the free meal.

"Where did *that* come from?" John asked.

"My pagne," I said, looking at the folds of the green and blue cloth I still held around me, suddenly aware that something else might be lurking inside. "I think I'll wear pants today."

I walked shakily back into the house, with John close behind.

"Wow, I've only seen giant scorpions when we've been repairing wells. How did it get in the house?"

"Don't know. As you say, they like dank places . . ."

"So . . . are we becoming dank?" John asked.

"More likely, with the lack of rain, they're being drawn to our garden."

"Like the snakes."

We'd so far killed two vipers and a cobra, all in and around our small vegetable garden and nyegen. We'd fashioned a spear from a knife strapped to the end of a long stick. It was not so much for killing as for coaxing the snakes from tight places, like cracks and holes in the walls. Once in the open, we pummeled the serpents with rocks. It was an awful act, but necessary. Due to our distance from medical facilities, we might not survive a lethal bite.

John and I took our time getting to the birthing house. It was so hot. We stopped by the clinic. There were no patients. Monique had her head in the medicine cabinet. Her greetings were muffled. The radio was fading in and out as it sucked the last of the energy from its cheap batteries. Medicine vials littered the desk, and Basil sat on the floor playing with an empty one. I was a little surprised to see him. More and more she left him with Blanche as he refused to stay on her back and wanted to get into everything. He glowered at us under furrowed brow.

"Fatumata, before you go, we must speak of the women's field," she stepped closer, resting her hands on the desk. "If God wishes it, the rains will be falling heavily soon and we must plan for the growing of baby food. We must wait until everyone has planted their own fields, then they will want to work in this one, especially if we have the seeds. Adama has secured a site for the field."

"Adama? I haven't seen him at all lately," I said. "Come to think of it, I haven't seen Dramane either."

Neither of them had been playing the nightly belotte.

"As for Dramane, he has left for the Ivory Coast. To find money . . ."

Well, he hadn't gone after Korotun. She was safe from him at least.

"Adama is around, and has found a field for the women."

"Okay." I eyed her suspiciously. "And it's a good one?"

"Yes, yes, Fatumata," she said. "He has done a good job this time. The dùgùtigi made sure of it. The field is big: 1.5 hectares. And the head of the women's group in each quartier has been able to gather enough beans, one gourd from each family, to plant. And the village will pay for the purchase of peanuts."

"Has it been plowed yet?"

Each of the four quartiers was responsible for plowing their section (done by the men) and planting it (done by the women).

"As for the plowing, the women say the men will do it."

"And," John said, "I plan to work with Daouda on digging the medical waste pit soon. Then you will have a place to throw your trash."

"Ah, I am becoming a professional," she said, straightening her blouse and wiping imaginary dirt off her forearms. "Monique, the professional." She laughed heartily and went back to her organizing. John and I continued to the birthing house. I found myself peering into the crevasses and crannies of the walls, looking for a twitch or reflection. I imagined scorpions were watching my every step.

Within the week Daouda was digging the medical waste pit. The ground was as dry as old bone and as hard as ledge. It was long work, work that Daouda had done for years. Almost all the villagers were in good shape, since their lives depended on physical labor, but Daouda's body was that of a god. Ropes of muscle made up his legs, arms, and neck and coursed down his back in a perfect V. His hands were like the rocks he pried from the ground. It seemed perverse that men in the U.S. would pay untold thousands of dollars doing rounds on machines to look like the average Malian villager. Daouda had dug the hole so deep I could no longer see his head when he stood up inside it. John lowered and hauled up buckets of soil and stone. Behind them, the clinic door was open and Henri watched them from the opening.

I sat down on the front porch. I was writing a progress report on the birthing house, careful not to make mistakes that the ditto paper would duplicate. Tedious. I ran my fingers through my hair, twirled the ends, and thought about how long it had been since I had had a haircut. A distraction.

Out came the scissors and two-inch mirror, which I perched on a chair against the metal porch post. I wet my hair and began to snip. I had to be careful. I didn't think that John would take a shining to a bowl cut, and my wavy hair could easily look just plain poufy, like a dandelion gone to seed. No matter how I contorted, I could not see and cut the back part. I struggled with various angles, elbows out, bent over, forehead thrust forward. Acting with blind faith, I thrust the scissors into my thick hair in hope of imposing some symmetry on the unruly thatch. As I watched the clumps fall to the floor and twisted my head to attack the other side, I saw a pair of feet, Monique's feet. I hadn't even heard her approach.

I looked up from under my bangs. Monique had one hand over her mouth, and another gripped the post like she was trying to steady herself. Her eyes were huge, and wet. She took a small stumbling step forward, her hand clenched and unclenched as it released the post and seemed to search for more support.

"Monique, what's wrong?"

I dropped my scissors, stood up, and put out my arm.

Her dark eyes squeezed closed, reopened and a flood of tears rolled down her cheeks. I saw her mouth move behind her shaking hand, but there was no noise. She fell into me.

"What's wrong?"

It took all my strength to help keep her up. My mouth had gone dry with fear. Goosebumps spread over my arms.

"What's wrong?" I almost screamed.

She reached for the door to the house, drew it open, and slid along the wall and inside, finally falling onto the white bench by the table. Her head dropped and her face disappeared into her palms.

"I heard his name. His name. His name," she said in a hoarse whisper.

"What?" I asked as I sat down beside her on the bench.

"His name, on the radio. His name."

Oh no. Pascal.

Monique was silent, and then she moaned as her grief uncoiled. As if the thoughts were too heavy to contemplate, her head fell between her legs and thrashed back and forth. She looked like she was sinking. Monique shuddered and sobbed, and I felt the warm tears on my ankles. I had never seen anyone cry here. I didn't know how to comfort in this culture. I longed to gather her to me, to hold her. Awkwardly, I wrapped one arm over her shoulders and back, firm and present. As I felt her body rock and quiver beneath me, silent tears fell from my own eyes.

I held Monique as the drifting lines of sun and shadow passed over our bodies and the day edged into afternoon. Crying was punctuated with wails that ebbed into profound quiet spells. We sat until the ebbs grew longer, until she became as still and quiet as sleep.

I lifted my arm. Monique sat up, straightened her back, wiped her swollen face on her pagne, and finally turned her face toward me. Her skin glistened, but did not glow. The deep reds of her complexion had gone blue, only a moist crimson rimmed her eyes. Her lips trembled for a moment, and then settled into her firm, clenched jaw.

"His name was announced on the radio today. He was on the border of Liberia. A skirmish broke out. He was shot. It was over, like that."

She grimaced. She splayed her fingers and looked at the empty space surrounding the one that had lost the ring.

"Fatumata, what am I going to do without him?" she whispered.

Her tears fell again and she quickly wiped them away and cleared her throat.

I shook my head. I had no ideas—nothing to say that seemed appropriate. I cringed at the thought of her never seeing him again, of sweet Pascal, lost forever. Why did this have to happen to Monique? Why now? Why was the only man she ever loved dead? We sat. We simply sat together on a white bench in the oppressive heat. My presence was all I could give her.

"Oh, I must go," she said suddenly. "Everyone must be wondering where I am. Look at the sun, I have been here so long."

"I'll help," I said, rising too.

Monique scooped cool water from the clay jar, washed it over her hands, wiped her face and shook, like a dog after a bath. Rewrapping her pagne and squaring her shoulders, she marched off the porch, then turned back to wait for me as I slipped on my sandals. Her face and stance betrayed nothing of today's events. Her life demanded that her grief reside within her. Outside these walls, her wound could never be revealed—the rhythm of custom and duty its balm and its cloak.

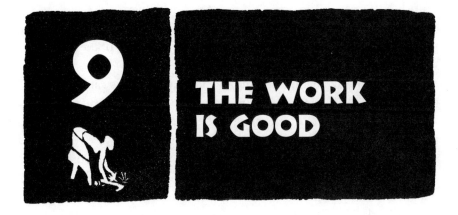

9

THE WORK IS GOOD

PASCAL'S DEATH CUT DEEPLY INTO MONIQUE, LIKE A FLASH FLOOD THAT HAD RIPPED THE LANDSCAPE. As I positioned Fousseni in the sling, I wondered if Mawa, or anyone else, noticed the change in her. Even if they did, they would never acknowledge it in public, any more than Monique would openly expose her pain. Here, among the familiar faces of the village, surrounded by the laughter and the motion of weighing babies, Monique attempted to project her normal care and enthusiasm as she chatted and listened. But her words and actions seemed as fragile as a brittle gourd.

In private, at our house, she cried. She visited whenever possible. Her eyes were continually red, and her face was puffy. At the family compound, her big fingers dawdled in her tõ, rolling the same ball over and over, never lifting it to her mouth. The loss of weight was noticeable. The angles of her body, her elbows, cheekbones, and shoulder blades, were pronounced and sharpened her features. Her hands and feet were dried and cracked, and the ends of her hair broke into a thousand filaments. I longed for her to lie fallow, untouched and unneeded for a season, to gather back her strength.

I awoke to the sound of random pings on the metal roof. At once I was grateful, there was rain for the fields at last. Then I was mad, as the birthing house was still open to the elements. By chance, today was the planned day to build the roof. We had received all the money we'd requested from folks in the U.S.; now the village had to hold up their end of the bargain.

John awoke too, and let loose a huge yawn.

"There's no way anyone is going to show up with this rain, especially not the Konés. As if they needed *another* excuse to not show up . . . Shit."

We walked out in the drizzle and I turned my face to the clouds. Despite the birthing house and John's scowl, it was invigorating. As we strolled the village, I could feel people's renewed energy as they headed to their fields. They did not look elated, but cautiously optimistic. It seemed ironic that one would wish so hard for something that heralded the start of the grueling fieldwork.

As of yesterday morning the materials for the roof had yet to arrive from Koutiala. Now more than ever the donkey carts were needed to shuttle between field and home. Lurching carts paraded in all directions, their wooden frames squeaking, but not one headed toward the birthing house. Indeed, when we arrived, the building was deserted. We called out greetings, hoping that a worker might be hidden somewhere, but there was no reply. The front door had been removed so that its wooden frame could be replaced, leaving a gaping hole like an open mouth howling for completion. Six bags of cement had been unceremoniously dumped on the front stoop.

"Oh great, if these get wet, they're useless," John said. "Let's get them into a corner, away from the rain. Maybe we can find something to cover them."

We dragged the fifty-pound bags into the front opening. Then John walked around the building to examine the work.

"Hey, the roof's here!" he called.

I went out back. The sheets of metal had indeed arrived and were laid on the ground, their corrugated waves looking like slices of cold sea.

"Let's check the bricks for the well, and the cover," John said.

"Aren't you scared?" I asked. My hands snapped like claws.

"Ah yes, the scorpions, my arachnid friends. You know, they seem to prefer the mud bricks. I've never found any under the concrete ones."

John and two young apprentices had made the bricks and well cover days ago, and now they needed to cure, to be kept wet, for at least a week so the concrete sufficiently hardened. The well itself was almost dry, yielding only muddy remnants good enough for watering the bricks and cover, but little else. John pulled off the straw that he had placed on the bricks to trap moisture.

"Looks good," he said, "They have been watered. A wet brick is a happy brick."

The bricks were substantial, about one by two feet, and angled on the ends so that they fit together to form an octagon. Soon, John and the team would excavate the area around the top of the well, place the bricks, and backfill. The circle of bricks would extend a couple of feet above the ground. A sloped curtain of clay covered in reinforced concrete would be built up around the well for drainage. Finally, the well cover would be placed on top. Villagers would still be safely drawing water from this well decades hence. We went to work, pulling water from the well until we heard the sound of a squeaky axle, and voices.

"Good morning," said the dùgùtigi.

A half circle of men stood behind him: Gawssou, Jean the mason, Kelemas, Dembeles, and even a smattering of Konés.

"As you can see, we have many people to help us today. Seven masons are here." He smiled proudly and pointed into the gathering.

I could barely believe my eyes. I gave a loud and indelicate "Wahoo!" with my fist raised in the air. John shook his head, and with a huge smile started shaking hands.

"Ah, the roof has come," the dùgùtigi said, looking at the side of the building. "The roof has come. It cannot be a birthing house without a roof."

The dùgùtigi turned back to the men and spoke in Minianka. One of the masons handed Gawssou a trowel, and Gawssou motioned us to follow. I looked at the gray sky. As long as the heavy rains held off a few more days, the birthing house would be completed.

We hunkered down on the tilled earth of the large communal field. It was a collective effort. The four quartiers were working at the same time in the same space, but each quartier was responsible for its own section of field. The Koulibaly, Dembele, and Kelema women had brought their own beans to plant, and we had evenly divided the purchased peanuts into four large equal piles. The Koné women had yet to show. Women were scattered throughout the field, planting, and bent at the waist. A few mothers sat in the shade of the large palm trees on the western edge, nursing their babies.

Their vibrant garments were the only color against the grays, browns, and dull reds of the earth, but not for long. Seedlings would soon have their fill of water, and put their newfound energy into leaves and shoots. Thunderheads would fill the sky, and sunsets would again be spectacular.

Mawa, the dùgùtigi, and Monique leaned over the earth, dàba in the right hand and small basket of peanuts in the left. They carved a small trench, and as they raised the hoe back in the air, they tilted their baskets just enough to flip a few peanuts out with their index fingers and thumb, drop them into the hole, and smooth them over with dirt. The dàbas dropped and the process was repeated. Again and again. They moved quickly down the field, planting their children's future in straight, even lines.

My wrist, however, had not mastered the graceful flick, and I dumped my entire basket. I left three peanuts, picked up the rest, covered the three with dirt, and tried again. Same result. John, on the other hand, possessed adequate fine motor skills and could perform the peanut-flick, but it required great concentration at the expense of straight rows. He meandered like a drunk, even once running into someone. Our performance was shamefully entertaining. The women chuckled and mimicked us. Monique was quiet, but she offered a weak smile when I looked her way. Now *this* was community. This was what I had imagined life as a Peace Corps volunteer would be like.

A half-dozen Koné women appeared at the field's edge. Their dàbas rested on their shoulders and their baskets hung in their hands. Pleased that they had showed up, and happy for the reprieve from planting, I made my way over to greet them and give them their peanuts, but to my surprise the pile was gone.

That's when the yelling started. The Konés pointed at the other women and back at the ground. The women in the field abandoned their task and came over, hands and arms jabbing the air. Monique and the dùgùtigi stood nearby and listened to what I assumed were expletives. John walked closer. There was more finger thrusting and raised voices until the Konés turned on their heels and made their exit. A moment of silence ensued before Monique and the dùgùtigi turned toward the remaining women. Monique thrust her index finger out and cocked her head from side to side, while the dùgùtigi held his hands in the air and threw out curt sentences. The women, thoroughly chewed out, returned to their work.

"These women here took the peanuts of the Konés," Monique said to me.

"On purpose?" I asked.

"Ah, oui, oui!" she said." The Konés refuse to plant even their beans until we find their peanuts, which are now planted in the other sections."

"One did not know if the Konés would show up. This is true," the dùgù-tigi said. "But does it help to take what is theirs? No, no!"

So much for communal utopia.

"So what do we do now?" asked John.

"Finish today's work," Monique said. "And then get more peanuts."

Within two hours we were finished. Women gathered their children and belongings and headed home. Elise walked toward us, wasted Karamogo on her hip. I thanked her for showing up and watched her depart. Monique had mentioned that Louis had finally found a fiancé for Elise, kid and all. She would soon leave for his village. After two years of trying to improve Karamogo's health, complete with the bra bribe, I had seen no change. Yet despite my frustration, I would miss her when she left; she was family.

John and the dùgùtigi went off to water the bricks as Monique and I headed toward the village in silence. Donkey carts and people made their way back between growing shadows, except for one figure coming toward us. The yellow-haired crazy woman. I hadn't seen her in months. I had assumed the curse of her infidelity had already carried her to a distant land. She flailed her arms and her head rolled from side to side, but it was not the dance of before. As she lazily waltzed closer and closer, we gave her a wide berth. Her ratty shirt swayed to the side revealing a grime-streaked belly, swollen and unmistakably pregnant.

What man would do that? Was this woman capable of consenting to sex? She probably had no idea that she had had intercourse, had no idea what was happening to her body, and would be unaware of what was going to happen. If she survived the torment of childbirth, what would she do with the squirming mass attached to her by a pulsing blue cord? Was that all part of the curse as well? And if the dùgùtigi was correct, and she had wandered here from afar, then she had no family to protect her. Her fate was left to providence.

We came to an open space close to the clinic, empty of people. Monique stopped. Her right hand caressed the empty spot where she used to twirl Pascal's ring.

"I miss him," she sighed. "I truly, truly miss him. Oh, how we could laugh together. Yee!"

She clapped her hands, and then brought them up to cover her face.

"My friend is gone, and I'm still here with le gars. Do you know what he wants now? He wants to sell my moped and buy a motorcycle. And do you know why? Because I cannot ride one. He knows my legs are too short. It is really too bad that he is Christian and poor. If not, he could take another wife and bother her rather than me."

"The idiot," I said.

"Oh, we fought this morning. I told him if he wants a motorcycle, he can find his own money. He takes all of mine already. Then he said that my health work and the money it brings will someday come to an end. I tell you this, Fatumata; if my work here ceases, never will you find me in Nampossela. It is for the work that I stay."

I knew she would not really leave. At least while the children were here and needed her. What mattered was that she felt powerful enough at this moment to say the words, to believe that if push came to shove, she could take the kids and go.

"I wish you could get away, take a little break. I'm sure the dùgùtigi would let you go, and he would convince Louis. Bakary and I can survive without you for a week or two. You need to go away and be surrounded by your family. Here, you are alone in your own head. You think too much," I said, echoing the words she had once said to me.

I held the newborn while I wove my way through the congested front hall of the newly opened birthing house, followed by the baby's grandmother, aunt, and mother. Women and children moved aside as best they could. The resting room was crowded as well. There had been a delivery yesterday, one bed was occupied, and bowls of food and clothing littered the floor. The grandmother and aunt moved in and carved out some space of their own, while the mother gingerly lay down on a firm mattress with clean gingham sheets and rested her head on the pillow. She looked up at the shiny roof as she moved her head in an arc from one corner to the other. I settled the child next to her.

"The work is good," the woman said, letting out a long breath. "You and Bakary did good work, Fatumata."

"Thank you, but it is the villagers who did the good work," I said, laying the bundle beside her.

John and I may have helped make this possible, but in no way did we take credit for the work. It was too easy to affix that sticky "white boss" label, and I rejected it.

The masons had finished in six days what had taken four months to organize. From afar, the birthing house was little different from all the other rudimentary buildings scattered among villages in Mali, but to us, it was spectacular. The light blue wash on the inside walls sparkled. The new unyielding iron beds were the pinnacle of comfort, the tin trunks, the acme of organization. Monique had nailed up health education posters from World Vision. All was fresh and welcoming.

Monique entered, hands washed, blood pressure cuff readied, and sat down beside the mother.

"Fatumata, did you know this woman has your name?" she asked.

"She is also Fatumata?"

"And also Dembele." she said, "Finally, Fatumata Dembele has given birth in my birthing house."

"Ah, this was such an easy labor for me. And look at my beautiful baby," I said.

"Oh yes, please take him," the other Fatumata said, smiling.

"Okay, I must show the baby to his father, Bakary."

I gathered the sleeping newborn and started for the door. The mother-in-law demanded in jest that her grandson be returned at once and threw herself with remarkable speed between the door and me. I resettled him next to his mother and waited for Monique to finish.

"All the women like it here, Fatumata. It is so comfortable. I cannot get them to leave," Monique said as we walked into the hallway. "All the beds are full. If I have one more birth, I will have to ask one of them to go."

We returned to weighing babies. It was much easier here than at the clinic, especially during the rains. The women had a dry place to wait, and they could stop by on their way to the fields. Mawa arrived with Lassiné and Fousseni. They were finally weighing in the green, healthy for their age. I loved to see the little creases in their legs. Folds meant fat, and fat was insurance against future illness.

"The dùgùtigi says bringing birth control here is good," Monique said as Mawa left. "But as you know, he has yet to embrace it for his own family."

"Yes, I know. Eight children and his second wife is pregnant."

"Yes. And he is still talking about a third wife."

I called in the next woman.

"I didn't tell you, Fatumata, but I played the cassettes of excision for the first time, for the family. They understood the information well, but we did not talk much about it afterwards. That will come later, with time."

I thought this was good news. Monique and I had decided it made sense for her, not me, to introduce the dangers of excision to the village. We felt it was too hot a topic for me to broach as an outsider. If this practice was going to be stopped, it had to come from within. It made sense that she started with her family before moving on to others. They were her easiest audience, and also her most important. With some talk, and a lot of luck, perhaps Gené could be spared.

With the dùgùtigi's eventual permission, Monique took her first vacation—a week with her uncle and aunt in Segou, a city two hundred kilometers to the northwest. Louis had been quick to say yes, after another of his daughters agreed to come from a nearby village to take over the household chores. As a woman and good cook, Monique would still be expected to work at her uncle's, but she would be away from the demands of the village and further away from those places that triggered memories of Pascal.

I missed her terribly. When the Konés put their last peanut seed into the earth, Monique wasn't there to celebrate the victory of the completely planted field. At night, when John and I ate with the family, she wasn't there to spice up Blanche's sauce or the family's conversation. And without Elise and Karamogo, the place seemed downright deserted.

At the clinic, I weighed babies with Henri. The women came and went quickly, not staying around to chat and learn, though Henri was doing a fine job. I was impressed with his knowledge. He had picked up a lot from Monique and seemed genuinely to care about the work. During a short reprieve near high noon, the most unexpected face peered through the clinic doorway.

"Good afternoon," said François.

He stood there for a minute, his dàba resting on his bony shoulder. He and Henri conversed in Minianka, and Henri handed him some aspirin.

"Fatumata," François said as he turned to go, as if what he had to say was an afterthought. I glanced up at his sun-framed silhouette in the doorway.

"I am going to build Monique a new kitchen."

"Oh," I said, then tried to hide the surprise in my voice. "That's very nice. She'll be very happy to hear it when she gets back."

Strange. I did not know him well, even after almost two years, and could not read him. But I sensed fear in him now, as he stood before me tense and motionless. Was he worried that she might not come back? Gené was in Koutiala with Monique's parents, and Monique had taken Basil with her. I felt certain that she would return but was fascinated that perhaps François thought she might not. Or maybe, maybe he actually missed her.

François lingered a moment longer, as if he wanted to add something, and then was gone.

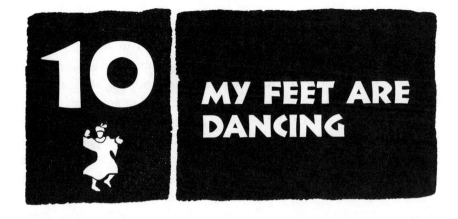

10 MY FEET ARE DANCING

"HOW DIFFICULT WILL IT BE TO GET A VISA FOR HER?" JOHN ASKED.

"Not too bad. It'd be different if she were a single male looking for work, but as a working mom with kids, the embassy knows she'll come back."

On a night this hot we would normally pull our bed outside, but approaching storms dissuaded us. The air ahead of the storms was densely humid and, coupled with the heat of the house, almost intolerable. Sitting or lying down was reason enough to perspire. Recently, John had taken to fanning himself to sleep. Now, he abandoned the foam bed altogether and lay on the relatively cool concrete floor, naked.

"Hand me the fan, please," he said.

I felt around and couldn't find it, so I turned on a flashlight. A large spider, a *cèkòròba yuguyugu* (old man who shakes), scurried into a crack of the termite-eaten window frame. The wind picked up, lifting a corner of the metal roof.

"Looks like we will have to put more rocks up there to keep the metal down," John commented.

I tossed him the hand-held straw fan, and switched us back into darkness. Distant flashes lit the window slats, and drums of thunder rumbled past. A few heavy drops hit the roof.

Just as I couldn't stop the weather from eroding my new house, I couldn't stop time from carrying me away. In less than two months, my time in Nampossela would be up. I was not ready to say good-bye, not just to the people, but to the lifestyle. I cherished spending almost all my time out-of-doors, taking bucket baths under the stars, watching thunderheads pile the sky, and walking and dancing by moonlight. I loved living in an inviting community, where you were always asked to share food and drink, where you spent time greeting and joking rather than avoiding others because of a busy schedule. Generations intermingled, there was always an excuse for celebrating, and death was sad, but not feared.

In the end, John and I had decided against extending our service another year. We were tired of the heat, of bountiful tŏ, and of being ill. Looking back, we had been sick, or at least under the weather, about half of the time and didn't relish the idea of another year of pumping our bodies with harsh drugs to keep malaria, amoebas, and other parasites at bay. We longed for a vacation, six weeks in Greece and Egypt, before flying into New York before Thanksgiving. And our friends and family were ready to have us home.

But leaving Mali meant leaving Monique, and that was a thought I couldn't stand. I wanted to invite her to visit us. After being host to us for two years, she could come and see our country, with us as hosts. Next April, six months away, seemed like a good time, not too cold in the U.S., and not yet the rainy season here. I had no idea how long she could be away, but a month seemed enough. John and I knew that we'd have to ask the dùgùtigi's and Louis' permission before we asked Monique, and we had a plan. Monique could teach Henri the essentials of operating the clinic and performing prenatal consultations. The old midwives could attend births at the birthing house, or women could go to Koutiala. And one of Monique's younger sisters could come out to cook and clean for the family. It would be an extra burden for everyone, but when would Monique have this chance again?

Luckily, the dùgùtigi was ecstatic at our proposition, viewing Monique as Nampossela's first ambassador. And Louis was amazed, asking questions about what she would see and do. Though he worried about not having Monique around, he found a month tolerable. François said only that he would like a gift from America, and stared straight ahead. Thus, permission was granted.

Monique returned from vacation refreshed. I barely saw her before she was once again attending births. It seemed as if the women had postponed their labors until Monique came back. A month-long trip to the U.S. could make for a lot of overdue babies. I told her to come out to our house when she was finished, no matter what the hour; I had something to ask her.

It was after 11 PM when she showed up, but I wasn't close to being sleepy. It was a refreshingly cooler, stormy night, with wind shaking the palm tree fronds like giant rattles. John and I sat inside. Monique took a seat, and we provided Basil with a couple of tin cups that he took to banging and stacking in between trips to his mother for sips from her mug. We told her of the success of the communal field and of Henri's growing capabilities and confidence at the clinic. She told of her time away.

"I think that I will be okay now," she said. "I thought about many things when I was away."

"The idea was for you not to think."

"What I want to say is that I thought in different ways. It was very good. I saw that I have my work and I have my children. And as for my marriage, that . . . pati, you know, ever since my return, le gars has been treating me nicely. He said he missed me. Me, I think this cannot be true. He gets along with me for the moment, but I know that in a few days it will start again. You see, if we are not together he misses me, but me, I have never missed him. But I did miss you. I don't know what I will do when you leave."

"Well, actually, Bakary and I have something to ask you about that."

I glanced at John, who was looking ridiculously eager.

"Would you like to come visit us in the U.S., after we have left? For a month next April, to visit our villages and the big cities?"

"Visit you in the United States? Really?" she asked and looked up at the ceiling. She was silent for a long time before she spoke.

"Yes, Fatumata, yes, Bakary. If you wish it, then I will go."

She looked me in the eyes, then hung her head down and took a deep breath. Her hands were folded tightly in her lap. I wondered if she didn't believe us. Many people here dreamed of going to the U.S.; it seemed the Malian equivalent of winning the lottery.

"Monique," John said, "we have already gotten permission from Louis and from the dùgùtigi for you to go. It's okay with them."

"*D'accord*," she said, her severe expression unchanging.

Maybe I had misjudged her. She didn't want to go. We sat. We sipped our Ovaltine. Basil played with the ends of the straps that tied our cushions to the backs of the chairs.

"Monique, what's wrong?" I asked, tentatively. "If you think the women cannot spare you for so long a time, maybe you could come for ten days or two weeks."

"No," she said, "It is not that. It is just that I don't know if I can hold on that long. I have only ridden on a motorcycle once, with Bakary to Koutiala, and the longest I have been on a moped is two hours away from Nampossela, for a birth."

"What does that have to do with coming to the U.S.?" I asked.

"You said that you were on a plane longer than ten hours. I have seen planes pass in the sky. They are so, so high up. I don't think I can hang on so long, so high."

A picture flashed through my head of Monique straddling the slippery top of a plane, gripping two small handles, her hair whipped back by the wind, and her knuckles cramping. Somewhere off the coast of Nova Scotia, I yell for her to hang on just a little longer . . . you're almost there. I began to laugh.

"Wait, wait Monique! You don't ride on the outside of a plane. You ride on the *inside*, like a car. There are seats and windows."

"Inside?!" she asked, looking at me, then John, who was also laughing, then back to me again, "you ride *inside?*"

"Yes," John said. "They even have televisions, bathrooms, and serve you food."

"Okay, then I accept your invitation. Yes, yes, yes, I will come, I'll ride on the inside."

Then we had the conversation I had dreamed about. We talked about what we would do and see. I pictured her visiting our national museums, sipping coffee at a sidewalk café, and grocery shopping at my hometown IGA. For me, it was the only way I could leave Monique, knowing that I would see her again, that I could share my world with her. It made my leaving feel less like the end of the line, more like an arc of an unfinished circle. I knew she felt the same, for she had said yes, even to riding on the outside.

"Fatumata, what are you going to show Monique in your country?" asked Oumou, bringing her daughter up for weighing. Heads turned when she spoke, despite her shy whisper. I placed the infant in the sling, careful to support her head. At almost six months old, she was on the small side, but healthy. With birth control on its way, Oumou was hopeful that this would be her last child.

"Well, I am going to show her my village, in the countryside. And she will also see the big cities."

Murmurs of "Bamako" traveled around the group of women.

"Yes, like Bamako, only a lot bigger and taller."

How could I explain the unearthliness of New York? The lights, the traffic, the miles of asphalt and steel, the rush of people, cars, and subways?

"And we will make presentations to people and tell them about this wonderful country of Mali, and the village of Nampossela."

"And I," Monique said, pointing to the left side of her mouth, "I want to see one of those doctors you told me about. Some nights I scream in pain from these teeth. Now both sides hurt, especially when it is cold. I want to see one of those doctors. And I want to see the ocean."

Word of Monique's trip had quickly spread, and the women were exceptionally animated today, asking her all sorts of questions in Minianka. Monique spoke and gestured, eyes wide, head turning this way and that. The entire clinic porch had stopped in hushed and attentive silence. I could tell she was explaining the plane ride, due to her use of *avioni*, the French-inspired Bambara word for plane. Her hand motions shot up into the sky, floated, and came barreling back down. From her explanation, I gathered that Monique thought the plane took off like a rocket. I'd have to clear that up later.

The rare and intrusive sound of a motorcycle floated over the wall, heralding a stranger's arrival. We could hear it making its way toward the center of the village, in the direction of the family's compound, revving and slowing at the many turns. Louis opened his eyes; Blanche put down the pot she was scrubbing; Monique came out of the cooking hut, slatted spoon in hand; and John and I stopped chewing our tõ. Basil let go of the baby goat's tail, and the kid ceased bleating and twitched its ears. Visitors always brought the unexpected. The sound came closer and closer, until the motor cut off outside the compound door.

"*C'est lui. C'est le patron*—It is him. It is the boss," Monique nodded. She sucked in her breath and walked back into the cooking hut.

"Aw ni su," came the greeting, and then the man.

Mr. Mariko had arrived! He was decked out in his government official's best—a pressed blue shirt with large lapels and matching blue pants, tailored to fit. I had only seen him behind his short, trim desk in his small square office; I didn't realize just how tidy he looked until seen in the uneven, organic world of the village.

"I ni su," rang the communal reply, with Louis' husky voice joining late. He was trying to shake off his millet beer-induced nap.

Mariko strode around and shook hands, hovering over Louis to exchange the longer greetings that befit an elder's status. Blanche retrieved a special carved sigilan and, with a curtsy, placed it on the ground. He ignored it for the moment, stood in the middle of the compound, and spoke.

"I have come and have something to say."

"Shall we go to see the chief?" I asked.

"No, no, please bring him here. And the village secretary, Adama, too."

I hadn't thought that the meeting would occur here, in our own compound. The whole family (except François, who had already made his exit) would hear what was being said, but maybe that was intended. The chief was asleep, just inside his hut, but jumped at the news that Mariko had come. He donned his hat, washed his face with water, and offered to get Adama himself. I readily agreed and returned to the compound to wait.

Evening gave way to obscure night. The family became recognizable only by their silhouettes. Monique left, empty basin on head, to get water at the pump. John sat by Mariko, making small talk about motorcycles and beans. Blanche shuffled about, gathering two small iron bowls connected with spikes. She filled them with karité oil, set a long piece of cotton in the oil, and then lit it with a gleaming ember. She stuck the lamps into the walls above us where they flickered, casting fluttering shadows.

I kept looking at my watch. Finally, the dùgùtigi came in. Adama soon followed, clad in a crisp shirt, suit pants, and faux leather shoes, not his usual village attire. He greeted Mariko with the utmost respect and formality and took his place near the chief. Blanche withdrew just beyond the dim orbs of lamplight. Mariko leaned forward on his stool, with outstretched hands.

"Greetings to you and thank you for receiving me tonight. I have come to your village of Nampossela from my village of Koutiala. Though we are not from the same village, we are all people here. We are all brothers and sisters, and as such, we must look out for one another. I have come as a representative of the health workers of Mali to talk to you, dear colleagues and friends, about the health program in Nampossela. The health program you have here is an extension of our national program; it is meant to improve the basic health of the men, women, and children of our country."

He paused, hitching up his pressed pants.

"Monique Dembele is the primary person responsible for carrying out this national initiative in Nampossela. She is here to attend to the basic health needs of your people. She is here to give you advice and medicine, to help women through childbirth, to take care of the infants and children. In return for her service, she receives a salary, as does each and every health worker across Mali."

I noticed he was looking directly at Adama and the dùgùtigi, both of whom were looking intently at the earth. They added a polite "Uh-hum" whenever Mariko took a breath or had a pause in his speech.

"Under our national law, the person salaried is the only person who can claim his salary. It is this person's signature that must be on the receipt we send back to the government. This is our law. We have a range of salaries for our health workers in Mali. While they vary according to the worker's seniority, experience, and training, we do have a minimum salary that we pay to most village-level health workers. The lowest salary that we offer is 15,000 CFA per month."

Monique had always received only 11,500 CFA. Who knew if Adama was pocketing the money himself or using it to cover other village debts? All I knew was that Monique had worked for every last CFA. I stifled a gleeful hoot with my hand—she had just gotten a raise. I glanced at Adama, but could detect nothing in his demeanor.

"Aw ni su," Monique said as she emerged in the doorway, balancing the twenty liters of water on her head. She walked with heavy steps across the compound to a giant clay storage jar. Her face disappeared behind a cascade of water as she tipped and emptied the basin.

Mariko looked at Monique and then back at us. Monique made no attempt to join the meeting, but instead gathered cooking pots and eating bowls to be scrubbed, being careful not to clang them together.

"I trust I have said everything I came to say and have said it well," Mariko said. "We must work together for the health of our people. Thus I must request, as a representative of Mali's health workers, that Monique Dembele pick up her salary of 15,000 CFA starting this month. And should the village wish to train Monsieur Henri Traoré to work also as health agent here, and should you be able to pay for his training, he is most welcome to attend. Is everything understood?"

I felt like shouting for joy, and by the look on his face, so did John. But I also wondered if it was awkward for Monique to hear this, for her to be spoken about as if she was not present.

Louis nodded silently. Adama nodded once.

"Uh-hum. All understood," the dùgùtigi nodded vigorously and pushed his cap even further up on his head. Still looking down at the ground, he addressed Mariko, rocking his body forward with each phrase as if physically punctuating his sentences.

"Mr. Mariko, you came tonight to our village and we thank you. We have understood your words. We will inform the others."

Everyone stayed in place, talking of other subjects, waiting for the signal from Mariko that it was time to disperse. Out of respect, he would be the one to decide when the evening's gathering would formally end.

I did not feel like chatting. My mission was accomplished, and I no longer wanted to be a part of this man's world of meetings, showmanship, and decision making. I wanted to talk with Monique. I kept trying to catch her eye, but she avoided my gaze.

Finally, Mariko asked for the road. We all got up and walked him to the compound entrance. Following the good-byes, Adama vanished, Louis went back to his chair, and the dùgùtigi left to inform the old men. I thanked Mariko and told him I would be in touch if things didn't work out. He nodded, climbed upon his shiny maroon Honda Road Bike, and announced his departure from the village with the kick-start of his engine. It shattered the stillness of the night. A baby in the neighboring compound started crying. Then he waved good-bye and the red glow of his tail light disappeared around the corner.

John and I hurried back to the compound, anxious to see Monique's reaction. She was there as we had left her, bent over at the waist, scrubbing off burnt tŏ with millet stalks, the natural Brillo Pad. She straightened up as she saw us approach, quickly dropped the stalks into the pot, and raised her hand to slap mine in mid-air.

"Hey, hey! Fatumata! Bakary!"

"Yeee!" I said, slapping her hand, then grabbing her shoulders. John slapped her hands too and gave an awkward semi-hug.

"Pati, pati," her voice stuttered with astonishment. "Let me walk you home, so you can tell me what happened."

We acted out the entire meeting for her: Mariko's speech, the dùgùtigi with his relief that Mariko had come, Adama with his eyes fixed on the ground, staring out from his best poker face.

"And you just got a 3,500 CFA raise!" I said for my final point, or as Monique would say, *pointe finale.*

"Yuh! Ah, Allah!" Monique uttered throughout the reenactment, covering her face and shaking her head in disbelief and something I read as slight embarrassment.

"Bakary," she bellowed, as we fairly skipped back to our house. "Bakary, whoa, whoa, whoa." She was doing the "Volaré" song. "Now when I sing to you, it will be a rich woman calling your name."

John and I awoke to murmurings. He rose with a yawn, moved aside the mosquito net, and looked out the window and into the pre-dawn.

"It's the elders," he said, "all of them, sitting under the néré tree."

"Jesus," I said, donning a pagne. They were all there, the dùgùtigi and Gawssou too, sitting and chatting in hushed voices. I supposed they were doing their best not to wake us. I wondered how long they had been there. It wasn't yet 6 AM.

My eyes swelled with tears. Tomorrow we would leave, early in the morning, for Bamako. This was our last full day in Nampossela.

We hurriedly dressed and washed our faces. John went outside, while I used the bucket to pee. John's camel-like ability to hold in his morning urine still amazed me. I joined him on the porch.

John and I greeted each ancient man individually, starting with Louis. While clasping the elder's right hand, we heard his praise for our work, his wishes for a safe journey home, and for our return to Mali to be quick. If they didn't agree with the decision to give Monique her salary, they certainly didn't show it. We received blessings for a good marriage, for good work and health, and many, many children. *Allah k'an to nyogon ye:* "May God bring us together again." *Allah k'aw sàra:* "May God compensate you." *Allah ka a to an ka ninye:* "May God let us not forget what you have done." It took half an hour to cycle through the gathering. Then the dùgùtigi spoke, the elders listening, some at attention, some dozing off.

"My daughter and son, you will be missed. You have done good work. You have helped us to improve the health of our people and helped make Nampossela the model village that it is today. You came here, not knowing anyone and now you are one of us. Greet the people of the United States for us and do not take too long in returning here, to your village."

"Thank you, dùgùtigi," John said.

I looked at my feet, not saying a word. To speak would let loose a torrent. I simply nodded. It seemed like yesterday that we were moving through rows of chickpeas together and predicting twins. The elders slowly filed out, among benedictions, and "See you tonight at la fête." The party would be held in our honor and attended by the entire village.

"You will have your last meal with the family tonight," Louis said before he left. "We will miss having you eat with us."

He looked so old, I thought, as he slowly turned and walked away into the village. Gawssou walked part of the way across the field with Louis, talking, and then came back and stood by John and the dùgùtigi.

Gawssou lingered, took hold of John's hand, and swung it back and forth.

"Ah, Bakary is leaving soon," he said, smiling and shaking his head. "You must take me with you too. Me and all my children."

"Okay," John said. "Start getting ready."

"You will come back to Nampossela," the dùgùtigi said, a question etched into his statement.

"Of course we will," John said.

The dùgùtigi and Gawssou did not make their way to the compound door, but instead sat down on the porch. John went into the kitchen to the gas stove and boiled water for coffee and couscous, knowing their stomachs, especially Gawssou's, were never full enough. He mixed hefty amounts of sugar and powdered milk into both food and drink, and served breakfast to our friends with a mock curtsy. A man serving men. I watched as Gawssou pushed his cap back on his head and looped his dry, long fingers over the mug awkwardly, as if he had rare occasion to grasp handles. The dùgùtigi did the same. We were going back to a place where grasping handles was the norm, but where no one knew how to hold a dàba. John and I went back inside, to the piles of clothes, books, and assorted items that we had to go through.

"Some of this stuff we should give to the villagers," he said, "The worst of the clothes we should burn."

"How did we end up with four Swiss army knives?" I asked.

"Three are mine," he said sheepishly. "It's a be-prepared thing, left over from my Boy Scout days."

"Could you still 'be prepared' with just one? We should leave one for Julie."

Julie was the Peace Corps volunteer replacing me. (John's replacement would be living in Sinsina, a nearby village.) She would arrive to a well-stocked home, even if the roof was a little loose. A tinge of jealousy whipped through me as I thought of someone else living here, in my house, and working with Monique.

John went out to Gawssou and the dùgùtigi and presented them with the knives, then proceeded to show them what the various functions were. The men held their gifts in the palms of their hands as if cupping some precious creature. We took the opportunity to discuss Henri's health worker training. While in Koutiala tomorrow, John and I would stop by the hospital and drop off the money we had saved to pay for Henri's ten-month long certification.

Even François paid a surprise visit. He did not accept an offered stool, but stood awkwardly in the entranceway to our yard.

"Can you bring me back a cassette player?" he asked.

"A what?" I asked.

"A cassette player, a big one," he said louder and stepped forward. "From the U.S."

We agreed that Monique would return with one.

Monique came out to our house around noon. She had made us lunch, a rich peanut sauce over flaky couscous, with a sauce loaded with tomatoes, sweet potatoes, and cabbage. She had even fried and sprinkled with sugar my favorite snack: millet fru-frus.

I had a gift for her as well. The necklace made of freshwater pearls.

"Fatumata," she said and sat down hard on the chair, putting the food on the table and Basil beside her. "You are giving me this necklace?"

"Yes, remember the first time you saw it? You thought it was so miraculous, that these pearls had come from animals in water?"

"Yes."

Basil got off the sofa and his feet made an unfamiliar clack as they hit the floor. I looked down. He was wearing his first pair of shoes, courtesy of Monique's salary. I put the necklace on her, just like I had done that night when we first met Pascal. The three white strands glistened against her midnight skin like rows of shooting stars. We walked out to my motorcycle and looked in the tiny round rearview mirror.

"Ah, Fatumata. You know me so well."

Monique stayed for much of the day, letting Henri handle the clinic's patients. The dùgùtigi and Gawssou stayed for lunch, savoring Monique's cuisine. She knew we'd have guests. Their presence was their farewell. After lunch Gawssou and the dùgùtigi left for their fields, but Monique stayed on. Sitting on the porch with her, we remembered. The penis faux pas, the nights with Pascal, the births, the deaths, all the joys and sorrows we had shared together. And we focused on the future. We talked about training Henri, about when the birth control pills would arrive, and about all that she had to do to get ready for her big trip. She asked questions about Greece and Egypt, the Parthenon and the pyramids.

"Fatumata, before you go, I must give you my advice on marriage," she said. "You and Bakary will soon be fiancés, and I might forget to tell you this when I see you next. I do not have a good marriage, but I know what makes one."

She turned toward me and spoke slowly and deliberately.

"You must work little by little each day so you are not too tired on the day of your marriage. You must have fun this day. When you are married, you and Bakary must get along well. Do not fight. You should not do things that wear on Bakary. And Bakary should not do things that wear on you. Don't be afraid, Fatumata, I know Bakary will be very happy on this day. I hope that God gives you at least two children. And I hope that I will see them one day in Mali."

Night came swiftly as it always does when the day is not long enough. My senses seemed acutely aware, trying to absorb all the sights, smells, and sounds of this place, to better remember the paths, the homes, the faces, and the words.

Light from the waxing moon shimmered on the straw of the village roofs and washed over the ground. The heavy humidity of weeks past had broken, and the night was remarkably clear. The sky was clean. The rippled grunts of goats and foghorn bellows of cows merged with the murmur of human conversations. From the distance floated a melody of wooden flutes, punctured by an occasional shout. The musicians were gathered in the common to warm up, lightly striking the balafon and sounding the rich tremors of the djembe drum amid the squeals of the young.

"Are you ready, Monique?" John asked.

With a sigh, Monique piled the pots in a corner, covered the remaining tŏ, affixed her headscarf, and walked with us toward the door. Her pearls glowed yellow-orange in the firelight.

"Eh!" she said, and slipped her arm comfortably into mine.

"Blanche, Louis," I called inside the dark huts, "are you coming to dance?"

"Ohh . . ." Blanche said with a smile concealed behind her hand. "No, no. You go along."

Louis came out, stood at attention, and told us to enjoy ourselves.

"Fatumata," a voice called from a dark corner of the compound. François' angular face appeared into the light of my flashlight. "Fatumata, Bakary, you leave tomorrow?"

"Yes," John said.

"Remember the cassette player," he said. "*Bon. K'an b'u fò. K'a sira nyuman soro*—May you find the good road."

May you as well, I thought.

We walked out onto the path and Monique whispered, "Do you want to know the only thing he has said about my trip to the United States?"

"Something about cassette players?" I asked.

"Ah, this is all he can think about. He thinks they must be very large in the United States. I know the bigger it is, the more batteries it takes, and so he will never have enough money to use it."

As we approached the central square, we passed the belotte table, where Adama sat with his slickly outfitted buddies playing cards. Too cool for village dances, they wouldn't be attending, but rather would stay in the embrace of Western games and abrupt greetings. The young girls who surrounded the men slowly spun on their heels and uttered soft good evenings. Keeping his cards at his side, Adama stood and shook our hands, then just as quickly glued himself to his seat again. The others mumbled good-byes, and two breezily asked us to leave our motorcycles to them.

"Tomorrow is the day you leave. I think that it cannot be true. It will be a hard day, *de*," Monique said, adding emphasis.

She held her hand out in front of her as if admiring her fingers. She found a cuticle to pick. I chose to pull a loose thread from my sleeve.

The flutes grew louder, their sound flying above us like chasing birds. The balafon player ran his fingers through the notes as if they were children at play. Rising clouds of dust from stomping feet filled our nostrils. They billowed skyward, reflecting light against the deep azure night. It seemed as if all of Nampossela had emerged for the festivity: young and old, healthy and sickly, women and men. Groups of teens and preteens, dressed in their finest, glowed with anticipation and filled the square between the steps of the Catholic church and the courtyard of the mosque, not far from the fétiche house. Here, God in all forms kept watch over the energetic children and the relatively sedate adults.

Monique, John, and I gathered along the outside of the large circle and attempted to peer over the swaying heads of the bystanders and glimpse the dancers. I could just pick out Oumou in the sea of smiling moonlit faces. She was moving back and forth, hands out in front of her, clapping in rhythm with a group of women. She waved to us. Basil was grunting and struggling on Monique's back, wanting to be put down. She plopped him onto the ground and beside the densely packed moving feet and clothed knees. The mass was impenetrable. His face contorted in frustration, his cries drowned out by the music.

"Do you want to see, Basil?" John yelled.

He kept whining.

John hoisted him up and held him high. He squealed and yelled, his squirming finally settling down a bit as he became entranced with what he saw.

"Fatumata, Bakary," our names rolled and rustled through the crowd as people cleared a place for us.

"Yuh! Yuh!" A muscular boy called out as he walked the perimeter of the performance space and pushed the crowd back. A dancer needed his space. He jumped toward the stars, kicked out his feet, landed, and flipped out his legs again, each time sending himself higher and higher, beating the earth with his feet as he alighted. Sometimes the music seemed to follow his lead, flowing and conforming to the motions of his body, and sometimes he adjusted the rhythm of his leaping according to a subtle shift in tempo.

Within minutes, the dancing boy was spent and took to the sidelines, breathing heavily. His show was not in vain. Girls pointed and looked in his direction while talking to one another behind cupped hands.

Groups of girls clapped and two-stepped in unison until two broke into the middle. As the flutes played, they circled each other. If boys were a show of brute strength, girls were a show of poise and finesse. Their moves were less histrionic, but just as intense. Their footwork was rapid and smooth, like the wings of a hummingbird. They undulated their bottoms and shoulders in quick movements. Look at us, they mimed, look at us, they gestured in low bows before returning to their friends.

By now I had begun to dance in place. I walked forward to the rhythm and the crowd formed a space around me. Fatumata dancing was always a spectacle. I moved and jumped, waved and grooved. The crowd laughed and hooted, delighted. I looked at the circle, at John, holding Basil, and at Monique. I ran and grabbed her hand, pulling her into the mêlée.

The swaying crowd cheered wildly. I heard our names yelled over and over above the quickening beat. Monique tried to pull away, but was weakened by laughter. Her headscarf fell as she lowered her head to the ground, as if willing her feet to move.

And they did. Her long toes splayed, her feet pivoted on their heels, and then she shook, a stirring that extended up to her knees. She stayed bent at the waist, pulling so hard against my grip that, should I let go, she would tumble into the rows of onlookers. For a few seconds, the earth felt the tempo of her feet, and then, just as suddenly, they stopped.

Monique cackled, let me pull her farther into the fray, stood up with hands raised in the air, and called "Merci! Merci!" She had danced. In front of the whole village, she had danced.

We ran laughing, with John and Basil close behind, carving our way through the bodies, away from the circle of music. I caught my breath and Monique regained her composure, tying on her headscarf and tightening her pagne. John handed a stunned Basil back to his mother. How quickly we escaped the glow and frenzy. From the outside looking in, it seemed too confined to hold such energy. A gathering of people in a tiny village. A jubilant speck just south of the vast Sahara. I savored the feeling of being here, of knowing this place.

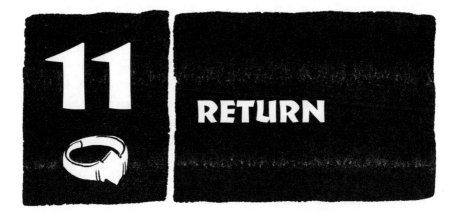

11 RETURN

MONIQUE ARRIVED AT JFK AIRPORT IN THE SPRING OF 1992, SIX MONTHS AFTER WE LEFT MALI. She had wanted to visit for our June wedding, but I convinced her otherwise, knowing how distracted and busy I would be. We spent almost a month seeing parts of America—New York, Washington, D.C., and central Ohio. I had worried that our friendship might lose its spark with her on my turf, that maybe our connection depended on the ingredients of tŏ and heat, but I was wrong. She, and our friendship, blossomed. I saw my world through her eyes.

The cities amazed her with their energy and size. She had seen Bamako, but nothing prepared her for New York City. She stared out the taxi window, amazed that the buildings just kept getting larger and larger. She went on her first boat, to Ellis Island, and stood at the foot of the Statue of Liberty. She walked the endless snaking aisles of grocery stores and pharmacies, overwhelmed by the amount and variety of items. She leaned her forehead against the glass at the top of the World Trade Center, looking down on a foreign world. So many glossy cars, and so many smooth roads. A huge world of perpetual motion. "Where are all these people going?" she wondered out loud.

She found Ohio the most gorgeous place she'd ever seen. She never imagined a place "so green with a ground so full of water." Farms of immense proportions, endless fields of waving grasses, and countless flowers in colors she had only seen on pagnes. She saw beauty everywhere—in the grace of ice skaters at an indoor rink, the pace of revolving doors, the light gurgle of water fountains, and the sweetness and softness of my family's golden retriever. "He is not a dog, but truly a person," she said. She marveled at the size of our refrigerators that keep so much food unspoiled and the dish and clothes washers that made our life so easy, "like having another wife." She loved cherry-flavored popcorn, whipped cream, strawberries, orange juice, and pizza. She dressed up, parading around Banana Republic in her first pair of pants, and posed in sunglasses and a fedora for my dad's camera. At her first (and only) amusement park, she "drove" an electric car around a track and screamed in terror riding the roller coaster with John.

She missed good rice, peanut sauce, and walking the village paths at night, remarking that Americans were never outside. And there was too much precipitation for her liking. Rains in Mali moved in, unloaded, and moved out, but here it could drizzle and bead the windows for days. "This is the true country of rain," she remarked, and yelled in glee when the sun came out in her second week.

Monique and I did many presentations (she speaking in French and me translating into English) about her health work—at schools, civic organizations, and churches—where she captivated audiences of all ages. She couldn't believe we had schools where they cooked for the children, and thought this was a fine idea. Over the course of three visits to Dr. Caldwell, she had over a dozen cavities filled and three root canals. The dentist charged me only his own costs and remarked that he didn't know how anyone could live in such pain. During Monique's first pap smear and blood test she decided not to test for HIV, as it was a death sentence whether she knew that she had it or not. On our last night together we looked up her horoscope. It said that she would never be satisfied with just one man, a revelation that mortified her in front of my parents.

By the time Monique boarded a plane to return, her hair, carefully braided by her sister-in-law before she came over, was loose. The morning light, flowing through the huge airport windows, caught the stray ends to fashion a glowing headdress. Monique did her best to appear happy. She repeatedly hid her face in her hands, then recovered, looking up to smile and wave as she moved away from us in line. "Good-bye and good evening," she yelled in English. I tried to appear cheerful and confident, to assure myself that her return was the right thing, that we would visit her soon and that distance and time would not diminish our connection.

Soon after Monique wrote:

Dear Fatumata and Bakary, hello,

This voyage for me, I have never had a voyage go so well as this one I just finished. When I arrived back in Mali everyone asked if I had become a black American.

Fatumata, your Dad asked me when I first arrived in the States what did I notice. I didn't know what to say when I was there, but now that I have arrived back in Mali, I know what to say. I smell the dust and the peanut sauce and the great heat. It is truly hot, just like you had told me. In America, I smelled the flowers, the humidity, and they smelled so good and I brought these odors on me here to Mali and I could smell them. When I was over there I didn't know that I had changed odors. But when I arrived back in Mali I could smell the odor and it smelled so good. I didn't want this odor to leave me. I smelled terrific.

Everyone is very happy with their presents. And the photos that I brought, they looked at the ones where I am wearing pants and they laughed and laughed. They had never seen a person like me in pants like that. The guy here, he loves his cassette player so much. Even if he has no money to put batteries in it, he loves it. He doesn't even like people to touch it. He looks at all the sides, and says "it is very good quality." I told you he is stupid and knows nothing.

Truly Fatumata, it is great nostalgia for me now. We will all pray to God to end this nostalgia. When I sit alone, everything comes into my head, all these thoughts. I don't know how I will live without you in this world. I am here in Mali, thinking about being there the day of your marriage even though I can't be. I greet everyone over there, without forgetting Brandy, the big dog.

Signed, Your Monique

Monique and I kept in touch over the next eight years through the exchange of long letters, cassette tapes, and packages. She wrote me of her burgeoning midwifery practice, and I told her of my studies and work in public health. In 1993, she had a daughter Christini, named for me. I read how this funny child was adored by her older brother, Basil, heard her singing and attempting English on cassette tapes, and kept pictures of her posed and serious, eyes twinkling with mischief. I sent Monique rubber gloves and medical scissors for her work, Tylenol for her parents, sequined shirts for her wardrobe, and toys for the children. In 1994 and 1997, after the midwife-attended homebirths of our two sons, Monique sent words of joy and congratulations along with small bundles of newborn baby clothes. Sewn by Apollinaire, they were made of bone-white cotton splashed with embroidered color; the shirts were short-sleeved and the pants short-legged. The tiny sets always arrived in the winter so were never worn, but they carried the same peppery-earth scent of her letters, a warm and welcome reminder of the life we shared.

In April of 1998, Monique wrote her last letter to me:

> I am pregnant. Fatumata, I didn't want this pregnancy, but God gave it to me. Ever since I gave birth to Christini, I have been taking the pill. I didn't have any problem with the pill until one day I was sick and went to the hospital and the people there told me to stop taking the pill. They said it was the pill's fault that I had back pain. You see? Now all is OK with my back, but all is not OK with my belly. Fatumata, if you can find a way for me to not have any more children, you could really help me. If not, what I am going to do? It is tiring. In any case, I am pregnant and I am looking for a way to rest. I am here, getting fatter each day.

I researched birth control alternatives—Depo Provera, Norplant, and tubal ligation—and wrote Monique of the pros and cons of each and where they might be available. She would have to go to Bamako. For tubal ligation, perhaps as far as Senegal or the Ivory Coast. I wrote that I wanted to return to help.

It was six months before a letter arrived from Mali. I ripped it open, wondering if she'd had a boy or girl, scarcely noticing that the handwriting on the envelope was not Monique's. The letter was signed by Maxim, her cherished cousin and a fellow health worker. I found the writing so graceful that the news slipped into me, as if he were giving a vaccination to a nervous village child, before I knew what had happened.

> 17 October 1998
>
> Dear Fatumata,
>
> The life of man is a succession of scenes. It is thus that at a moment given in your life, you came to know the land of Africa, our country Mali, far away from yours—the USA. It is here that you met my sister,

Monique. Monique was first a collaborator in your work, then more than that, a friend, a sister. God is the only master of this earth. He does to the earth and its inhabitants what he wants. It is thus that we, Apollinaire and Jeanne Dembele, parents of Monique; Maxim, Abel, Louis, Didier, Angele, Joseph and all our other brothers and sisters Dembele; the village community of Nampossela; François and his father Louis; and the children of Monique regret to announce to you the brutal death of our daughter, sister, and spouse Monique Dembele on the birthing table at the maternity ward in Koutiala on Thursday, October 15th, 1998, at 7:40 PM. The burial will take place on October 18, 1998 in Koutiala. May God accept her in his grace. Amen.

Maxim Dembele

John and I decided to return to Nampossela in the winter of 1999, after eight years away. We had to make sense of what happened to Monique—how could she, of all people, die in childbirth? What possibly could have gone so wrong? We had to mourn, to visit the hump of earth in Koutiala that marks her grave, and most of all, we had to encourage François to honor his wife's wishes and ensure Geneviève, Basil, and Christini attended school.

It wasn't long after our return to the village that I made my way to the birthing house. Maxim's letter was folded in my pocket, creased from a hundred readings, as I stared out a window. I let the sense of place wash over me—the wood-fire scent of the air, the distant pound of pestles, and the huddle of huts on dry ground pressed against the endless sky. I steeped myself in the feeling of being here. My visit was short this time: weeks, not years.

The massive birthing block, and the birthing chair that Monique and I designed, were gone, replaced by a worn birthing table. The wall was marked with a gray patchwork of concrete, where the slab had been torn out. Above it remained the large rough-edged discoloration, evidence of countless backs rubbing through the dull blue paint. The gray metal frame of the birthing table was scratched and chipped at the feet. The two black vinyl cushions, after bearing the weight of so many labors, dipped like plates. White mesh showed through the faux skin where the sides had been flattened by years of clenching hands.

Monique, my teacher, my friend, my sister. "Same mother, same father," as she once wrote to me. I could picture her here, wrapped in bright blues and sparkling gold, giving this room its only splash of vibrant color. A pregnant midwife, her large flat feet splay for balance as she leans over a woman in labor. Two bellies nearly touch: one pushing and one waiting. Her chestnut skin glistens in the stifling heat. In steady, fluid motion, her hands beckon another soul. Her dark eyes, warm voice, and sure smile give welcome comfort to another mother.

Four months ago, Monique's hands grasped the edge of a birthing table in Koutiala, just like this one, as if it were life itself. This time, she was the one giving birth. My eyes blink and my teeth clench. Oh God, I don't want to, but I can see her dying. Her palms crush the cushion, the insides of her fingers hook under the metal edge. She's uncomfortable and dizzy, her breath rises and falls. Waves crest with stifled howls that saturate the room. The force of a gale rips through from the inside. She pushes and groans. In her fading vision, the birthing table slants and falls away, swallowed by the rutted ceiling. She makes one final effort to heave the parcel of new life into the world. But instead, the moment passes, a dull and distant throb. Awash in an expanding sea of blindness, she hangs between two worlds. The light grays to nothing.

I loosened the scarf around my neck and hid my face in its wide band of orange stripes and turquoise suns. I knew sorrow's tears were not for public display, but it was hard to keep my eyes dry. I wiped my face, and noticed a storage trunk resting in one corner, vials and other instruments jumbled inside. Its lid hung off a single hinge like a broken limb. Cluttering the floor were used rubber gloves and wrappings. Monique never would have left the place in such a state. Koniba, the new midwife, was only in her second week of training as an apprentice when Monique died. She forged on as best she could.

I heard women talking in the nearby resting room. A newborn whimpered and was soothed back into silence. I walked along the hallway, past the room with the scale and blood pressure cuff, and peered in on two reclining mothers and their babies. The bed frames were rusted, but sturdy, and the foam mattresses looked like they'd been replaced. The mothers gave me tired smiles.

I twisted the silver ring on my finger. The skin underneath was already turning green. Flat, the ring broadened at the top to an irregular diamond shape, three etched lines on either side, matching the tribal scars on Jeanne's face. Monique died wearing this piece of junk jewelry on her left hand. Her family insisted I take whatever I wanted from her possessions. Would I like her favorite necklace? The one she wore on her last day? The freshwater pearls gleamed white against Monique's sister's dark pink palms. I swallowed hard. No, thank you. The ring was perfect.

My clay-colored dress stuck to me as I walked down the hallway and outside. I was unaccustomed to such intense and radiant heat, especially in February; there was snow on the ground back in Massachusetts. Being here felt at once overwhelmingly foreign and intensely familiar. The birthing house's façade closest to the ground had eroded down to bricks, but the structure was still sound. Still safe. I looked up to see the stenciled words, Mùsòjiginniso, almost unreadable, but still there.

"Looks good," John said, stepping onto the porch. Other than his untrimmed goatee and shorter hair, he looked much the same as he did eight years before. "The roof and walls are solid. No real termite damage. No holes or cracks. And the wells are fine, too."

A woman stood on one of the wells with legs spread for support. Her arms worked like pistons, hauling up a taut, quivering rope until a bulging *puissette* emerged. She flipped its contents into a large basin and tossed the glimmering sack back into the well. Two young girls stood by her, staring at us with large, dark eyes. John pointed to the smallest child who was now leaning against her mother's leg, bulbous bare bottom pointed in our direction.

"Amazing—diaperless. We spend hundreds of dollars each year on diapers for our boys. There are no diapers in Mali, and somehow... the country keeps going."

John paused, waiting for me to acknowledge his pun. I humphed and rolled my eyes. His grin broadened in triumph. I thought of Aidan and Liam, our two young sons, boisterous and blond, who were back home with my parents. It was strange to be without them, as if the years away from Nampossela were an imagination of mine.

A figure strode toward us along one of the main paths leading from the heart of the village. It was the dùgùtigi. From a distance he looked the same, with baggy shirt, pants, and wool cap. Only up close did I notice the lines in his face were etched deeper, and his temples and chin were peppered with gray. He stopped and stretched his back with a slight pained expression. Same maladies. Oh, I have missed him.

Against custom, the dùgùtigi looked into my eyes, as he had earlier that morning when we first arrived. I didn't think I looked that different, except that my hair was longer and I had lost some baby fat around the cheeks, but I felt self-conscious. I sensed that our presence made Monique's death more palpable.

We joined him on the path leading back into the village, stepping over chicken feathers and empty Nescafé packets. It was time to give Louis our sàya fòli (death greetings), a formal acknowledgement of Monique's passing, just as we had given them to Monique's parents in Koutiala the day before.

Gawssou caught up with us—blue hat, dancing eyes, vigorous greetings. He gripped John's hand all the way, as if letting go might mean John could vanish as quickly as he'd appeared.

"How did you find the birthing house?" the dùgùtigi asked.

"Good," I said. "I'm glad it's still being used. Monique wrote me that last year women from many neighboring villages were coming here to give birth with her, and have their prenatal consultations."

"Yes, everyone came to her. During the day, during the night, until 2 AM, 3 AM, no matter what hour, Monique worked here. Ah, but this midwifery work is very *hard*," he said, spitting out the last word. "She never rested, even after becoming pregnant herself."

The dùgùtigi shook his head and stopped to rearrange the straw on the roof of a granary and replace a few fallen bricks on a nearby wall. Into a crack someone had stuck the remnants of a blue plastic bag, string, and cloth. The dùgùtigi pushed the homespun patch deeper into the hole. He and Monique had cared for the village together. The dùgùtigi had guided the village, while Monique, young, but gifted in her mothering, had attended its future generations.

"After Monique's death," he continued, voice rising, "truly, the women cried, 'how can we live after Monique is gone?' The midwives in Koutiala, everyone around Nampossela, everyone cried this day."

"*Wadelay!*" he exclaimed, an Arabic word of surprise. "Ah, if you could have seen the crowd that gathered for mass in Nampossela after her burial in Koutiala. Oh, oh, oh, *oh!* There were so many people—animists, Catholics, Muslims—everyone came. And so many children. So many that she herself had midwifed. The villagers said 'Truly, we thank Monique. May God bring her peace in paradise.'"

He winced as he placed his hands on his hips again to stretch his back. As we moved through town, people emerged from shaded areas to greet us. Children were everywhere. That was nothing new, but I saw them differently now as a mother.

Young kids were the survivors of toddlerhood. They wandered about in packs of the same sex, not a parent in sight. Their independence startled me. I hadn't realized how we hovered over our children in the U.S. I searched the faces for Monique's son Basil. He was ten years old now. For a second, I even looked for his peers, for Karamogo's bony frame and little William's big forehead, before I remembered they were not among the survivors. Monique had written that William died of protein deficiency at the age of three, and Karamogo succumbed to illness on the eve of his fifth birthday. I did not look for Oumou or her children—after Daouda's death a couple of years back, likely of AIDS, they'd left the village.

Monique's daughters, Geneviève, now thirteen, and Christini, six, were both in Koutiala with Monique's parents, while Basil remained in the village. Monique wanted all of them to be in school. Though Nampossela now boasted a small school and two teachers, the chances of her children regularly attending classes without her here to support them were nil. Thus we hoped that Louis and François would give their permission and allow the kids to attend school in Koutiala.

Louis was dozing, limbs akimbo, in a hammock where the old fallen granary used to be. I walked quietly past him and peeked around the corner into the enclave. It was barren of people, animals, firewood, and other common accoutrements of a family. The only movement was of gray smoke lazily snaking out the blackened door of the cooking hut.

The dùgùtigi gently tapped Louis' shoulder and whispered in Minianka. I saw a glimmer of recognition in the cataracts that now blanketed the old man's eyes like wet scabs. He unfolded himself and struggled to greet us, seemingly lost in his blue robe, and finally succeeded in coming to a stooped-over position before falling back into the hammock. His angular face was gaunt and grooved, his skull pronounced. Something was missing that old age alone could not account for.

"Ah, Fatumata, Bakary," he said at last. "Welcome, welcome."

Louis' voice was as dry as chalk and his words slurred. I wondered if he'd suffered a stroke.

The dùgùtigi, John, Gawssou, and I sat down on the small wooden sigilans. I looked at the dust that temporarily clouded my feet. Everything was unkempt. Monique was the last woman to stir life into this space. Cancer had devoured Blanche three years earlier after two years of sickness and slow failing. Monique had written that Louis never recovered. Perhaps the hole I sensed in him was sheer loss.

Amadou Gakun was also present, recommended by Julie, the Peace Corps volunteer who came to Nampossela when I left. He would serve as our intermediary. I had almost forgotten we needed one. In important or delicate social situations, like death greetings, or proposing the children's schooling to Louis, an intermediary was expected. He did more than repeat our words; he served as a surrogate focus of attention. Here, where the outward show of grief was forbidden, he created emotional distance, allowing us to maintain our decorum. He was a thin, acne-scarred young man with large eyes, and he bowed slightly as he entered.

Louis, who had escaped the hammock, sat on the ground staring in the direction of the smoldering fire. Our circle was silent. John and I exchanged glances. It was time to begin, but François was missing. John gave a little shrug, and urged me on with a tilt of his head.

"Amadou," I said. "We would like to give our death greetings to Louis."

I directed my words to Amadou, who nodded and said "Uh-huh" after every few sentences as a sign that it was his turn to recite what I had said. He kept his gaze on the ground as his words and voice transformed my rusty Bambara into grace. "...Your difficult news found us. Our hearts cried. We know Monique is no longer here, but she is in a better place. We can't know her destiny, for only God knows it. We have come with gifts and greetings during this time of mourning. *Allah ka hine a la*—May God have pity on the deceased. *Allah ka ye fisàya ma*—May God put her in paradise. *Allah ka bila ka màra la*—May God put her in his kingdom in the sky."

"*Amina*—Amen."

Amadou's steady, comforting voice was like a balm over a raw wound. We presented gifts—soap, sugar, tea, money, and new clothes for the children—pulled them from our knapsacks and handed them one by one to Amadou, who passed them to Gawssou, who handed them to the dùgùtigi, then on to Louis. A gift to one touched everybody. Louis thanked us, and blessed us. The compound was again swathed in silence.

Later that day, I walked with Yvonne, François' eldest sister, toward the fields north of the village, along the dry bed of the sacred river, beyond the birthing house. Two boys sprinted past, rolling a hoop they urged on with sticks like an errant calf. François had a garden out here and he wanted to show us. Yvonne's caramel skin glowed in the late afternoon light. She was a large, regal woman who resided in Koutiala. Of all Monique's in-law's, she'd been the favorite, though she was responsible for Monique's marriage to François. Yvonne had been at Monique's side when she died.

"Ah Fatumata. This year, oh, how I have cried," Yvonne said. "I can't even do my sewing. Even to do my embroidery, sometimes, I get up in the morning, and just trying to prepare to do it I spend all my time crying." Her voice wavered and she looked away.

When she turned back her face was striped in tears. She wiped them away with her scarf, the moisture streaking the fine white cotton like trails of silver. Her honesty was unexpected. I was relieved. Like me, she could not always control her emotions.

"I miss Monique, too."

As I said her name, it was as if a buoyant darkness had been unsnagged and rushed toward the surface. I struggled to steady my voice. I kept my eyes on the spaces where my feet would land.

"Fatumata, I want to tell you about that day, in the maternity ward in Koutiala with Monique," she paused and touched my arm as we walked. I nodded and said nothing; I wanted to hear her story.

"Monique's mother Jeanne had fallen ill and could not be there, so Monique asked for me. When I arrived at the ward, I greeted her and we chatted. Her labor had begun the night before. In the morning, she came to the maternity ward and greeted everyone in the dispensary and visited the midwives. They told her, 'if it pleases God, you'll separate from your infant today. You'll give birth today.' Monique went to the market on foot to help advance the labor and then returned to the maternity ward. Madame Sano, the midwife, arrived around 6 PM. She said, 'Is this the midwife herself that is in the maternity ward today?' Everyone laughed. Even Monique said that she trusted this midwife.

"Madame Sano went into the next room to get dressed in her work clothes. Then she gave Monique a shot. The midwife came to me and said, 'Now, if it pleases God, maybe the labor will advance.' I went into the room next to her and then I heard Madame Sano ask Monique, 'Hey, Monique, what is this? You must have malaria, a lot of malaria.' Monique told her, 'Nevertheless, I've been treating myself for it.' The midwife called to me, 'Come take this, dump it out, clean it, and bring it back here.' I took the bucket; it held liquid that was almost green, liquid that had come out of Monique. After a few minutes I heard Monique making a funny whirring sound, 'Wwhhrr, Wwwhhhrrr,'" Yvonne made the sound with her tongue rapidly hitting the top of her mouth.

"She could breathe no longer. The midwife, she ran to me and said, 'Where is Monique's prenatal record?' We looked through her things and found it. The midwife said, 'Look at this person here, she has a lot of salt in her body!' Monique had the salt sickness. She ran back into the room. I no longer heard Monique making noises and yelled, 'Madame Sano, Madame Sano, come tell me what's going on!' She came out of the room. Then she went in again. Then she came out, and went in with another midwife. I went into the room. As I opened the door, I saw Monique lying on the table. She didn't move. Do you understand, Fatumata? I saw that she wasn't moving. The midwife said, 'This is what God has done, no one can refuse it. Thus, your woman has left us.'

"Oh, I tell you, Fatumata. All of a sudden, she was no longer living. It didn't even take a half hour. When she told me Monique was no longer there, I said, 'What am I going to do now?' I entered the room and I stayed at her side while I prayed. From 7 PM when she died, until 10 PM I stayed alone by her side. Then around 10 PM, the doctor came in. He operated on her to take out the baby. It was a boy."

Yvonne turned her head away from me again as she began to cry. I struggled to make sense of what she'd said. I couldn't believe the first time a doctor came in was hours after her death. What if her son had still been alive? Could they have saved him?

I'd spoken with Madame Sano in Koutiala two days ago. She'd seemed nervous talking with me, a white person from afar asking questions, but she, too, had given details about that night . . . Monique took Buscopan to calm the pain and another medicine to dilate the cervix early in the day, but her belly still hurt her, and she was not dilating. When the midwife examined Monique in the evening, she found that the liquid inside was green. Madame Sano thought that it could have been malaria, or it could have been meconium, signaling the baby's distress. Monique had a high temperature, a sign of infection or malaria, and no strength. She wanted to vomit, but she couldn't. She lay down and then started rolling around on the table. Then she fell into a coma, or as Madame Sano said, "began searching for the road to death."

Madame Sano had not mentioned the shot that she'd given Monique in her telling. It was probably a uterine stimulant such as Pitocin or Ergometrine, injections intended to control postpartum bleeding, but often used here to augment labor, something even Monique did, despite the hazards. Ergometrine, like methergine, was powerful and could be deadly if given to a woman who was anemic (as over half of Malian women were, due to chronic malaria) or had high blood pressure. A high dose could cause a heart attack or stroke. I had seen Monique's prenatal chart and knew her blood pressure had not been recorded. Her brother had mentioned that Monique had dizzy spells during her pregnancy, a sign of anemia or toxemia (pregnancy-induced high blood pressure).

My desire to pin down the hows and whys, to place blame on something or someone, was overwhelming. Yet I realized that there was, in both Yvonne's and Madame Sano's stories, a sense of calm in Monique's final minutes, a lack of urgency in the actions or in the telling. That was a sharp contrast to the flurry of activity to prolong a life in our country. Hers was not seen as an emergency, but rather as the hand of God. How much of this attitude was the product of simply not having the knowledge or resources to save the dying, I didn't know. I did know that I had to accept their stories, for they were all I had.

I told Yvonne how we received the news of Monique's death by letter. I told her of the details of that November day. Of how we held our boys next to us and cried, not wanting to call our families because to do so would confirm the news. Of the irony that my last letter to Monique had discussed birth control methods and the possibility that I could return. Now I had come, after all these years, and Monique was not here.

We were silent, our footsteps crunching in the sand the only sound. I let the quiet come, knowing it was not awkward here. We approached the garden. The crop fields yielded nothing but broken stalks this time of year, but the garden was fecund, fragrant, and thick with life. It was at least a half-acre. Saturated scent tumbled off banana tree leaves as broad as a man's back. Papaya branches proudly displayed their grooved, green ellipses of fruit. A wall of leafy plants hugged the garden's enormous chain-link fence. We paused in front of the metal gate.

"You know, Fatumata, she and her husband did not get along. Not too long ago, I went to her husband and said, 'If you don't want this wife then we will separate you. I will no longer be your sister; you will no longer be my brother.' But he continued to mistreat her." In a low, heated voice, she added, "When Monique knew the birth would be soon, she went to leave for Koutiala. But there was a problem. Her husband did not want her to go to Koutiala for the birth; he wanted her to stay in Nampossela."

"And give birth with whom?" I asked.

"Alone," Yvonne whispered. "He said that she was a midwife, she could birth herself. He would not take her to Koutiala, so she was forced to find a ride."

Monique's prenatal chart showed that she hadn't started prenatal care in Koutiala until her seventh month of pregnancy. Getting into Koutiala had obviously been difficult. Even so, I was stunned—to give birth alone, in this land of community, was unthinkable. So many factors seemed to play a role in Monique's death. The shot in labor, a misuse of Western medicine, was likely one cause. And so was the subsequent lack of emergency care to save her or her baby. And so were the myriad possible problems leading up to her death: anemia, toxemia, malaria, lack of prenatal care, exhaustion from a job where she was overworked and underpaid, François' refusal to bring her into town or otherwise support her, and the burden of being pregnant when she did not want another child. There were so many reasons. Take one or two of them out of the picture, and she might still be here. I thought, desperately, selfishly, that if only she had stayed with me in the States, and had never come back to Mali, she might be alive today.

From inside the gate a figure emerged and spoke. François had his father's voice, deep and rough, but one that somehow found its way from thin and seemingly unmoving lips. He wore a child's white winter hat with the chinstraps tied up over his head in a bow, and a blue polyester jacket. He nodded to Yvonne, and then turned toward me.

It was all I could do to keep from screaming accusations. Yvonne's revelations rung in my ears. I looked at her. She smiled, as if our earlier conversation had been as light as millet chaff. I thought of Geneviève, of Basil, of Christini, and focused on what was most important. We needed François' support. My exchange with him was short and perfunctory, the bare minimum required.

François did an about-face, glancing back over his shoulder, and told us to follow. The garden was impressive. In addition to the chain-link fencing there was a pump for water: true luxuries here. The dried thorny branches most often used to fence out roaming ruminants required constant repair. And drawing water from the depths of a nearby well was a tiring and perpetual task.

François pointed to plants, telling us their names in French. We marched between lines and lines of lettuce, rows of bulbous green peppers, and hot peppers like exclamation points, Rubenesque eggplants, and crisp cucumbers. And fruits: in addition to banana and papaya, there were oranges and guava. The rows were well planned and mulched, making careful use of sun and water.

I looked out along the garden's border where the emerald green of this satiated parcel met its russet, thirsty neighbors. I'd never spent this much time with François. Despite this stroll through Eden, there was a vast desert of unspoken words between us that I could not cross.

Back at the guesthouse, I retrieved the key the dùgùtigi had given me, walked into the antechamber, and then opened the room in which we were staying. The scraping resonated off the tin roof and barren walls. On the floor were our travel bags, the only objects in the place besides two mattresses on worn, squeaky frames, and a kerosene lantern with smoke-blackened glass. The beds were heavily stained and friable, deposits of foam layered the floor. The walls' yellow paint had faded to blond and there were streaks of rust beneath the iron-slatted windows.

"I don't care what the Michelin guide says, I only give this place two stars," John said, bouncing on the creaky bed. "Hard to believe you lived here for six months."

"It had a different feeling then."

The outer door clanged open and a group of dirty, smiling, scrawny boys entered. One had an injured bird in one hand and a slingshot in the other. The creature's eyes bulged and blinked, its wings pinned back by little fingers. The boy was nonchalant about his snack, more interested in us. I understood that the children were hungry here, but I still hated to see animals suffer.

"Basil," John said.

I looked up. The crowd parted and Basil, long and thin with unkempt hair, huge eyes, and a tentative smile, came forward. He was wearing a T-shirt that we'd sent to Monique last year; it read *Police Chase 5K, Newark, Ohio.*

"Hello, Basil, how are you?"

"Peace," he whispered.

"Come over here," John said, beckoning him closer. "Come see what I've got."

Basil said nothing, but moved next to John, who pulled his sketchbook and drawing implements from the knapsack. Basil stared, enraptured, as John began to draw the head of a young boy who was leaning against the doorframe. John elongated the nose and added a goofy, toothless smile as Basil laughed into his hands. Other boys jostled for a peek. John feigned ignorance, erased his mistakes, added a bird beak, and the game went on. I was delighted and surprised at the ease between the two, though I should have expected it—John played this way with our boys.

I sat back and watched them, thinking of Monique and how she'd never met our children. I remembered how excited she'd been when she heard I was pregnant with our first:

> I am so happy to hear that Fatumata is pregnant! Thank God. I hope that this child comes with great pleasure into the world. I will keep praying for you always, because when you are pregnant, you are always tired. Truly Fatumata, I know how you are feeling.
>
> I hope God helps you, as I cannot go over there to help you. I wish I could though. I thank the midwife even before the day of your birth. Fatumata, don't worry. It will pass quickly. It is tiring, but it passes quickly. Have courage, Fatumata. All the families here are happy about your pregnancy and they want to see this child.
>
> Bakary, I know you are ready to be a Dad! Good luck. You must do everything for Fatumata now. You must give her everything that she needs; if not, I will come and beat you. It is you who must cook for her now, right? Yes. You must cook the very best cuisine ever.
>
> Here are some clothes for the baby. Yvonne did the embroidery. Fatumata, I wish that once the baby is born, you carry him on your

back with this pagne. You take a photo and you give it to me. I really want this. Jeanne said she would love to see you now, pregnant, but it is not possible. Anyway, she just wants to laugh . . .

Our boys would never know Monique, other than through our recollections. But her children still had a chance to know us. I wondered if Basil had heard of our hopes for him to attend school in Koutiala.

"I'd like to take a photo," I said, and shook my camera. "A photo."

I looked through the smudged lens and the ten boys instantly put themselves into kung-fu poses, jostling each other. The dùgùtigi appeared in the doorway, and we offered him a seat. John handed him the small photo album of pictures we'd brought with us.

"It is good to see your sons," he said, lingering for a moment on an image of our two boys, clad in winter coats and impish expressions.

The dùgùtigi offered to walk us to dinner. The boys disbanded, taking different paths. Basil waved a small good-bye and disappeared around the corner, alone. We headed in the opposite direction, away from town, toward the new quartier. We passed our old home, now inhabited by one of the schoolteachers. The dùgùtigi proposed a tour inside that John and I politely refused; we'd like to remember our house as it was. Behind it was another teacher's home, where we would dine. Eating here made sense from the dùgùtigi's point of view; the teacher was Malian, but like us, from away and respected simply because he was a guest. With Monique gone and our old host family decimated, we took our meals outside the village.

The sun went down and the night was once again free to embrace the land. Two lights bobbed in the distance and the hum of an automobile engine vibrated across the field. John and I watched as a small truck puttered past.

"That is Kelema, the blacksmith. He has done well. He also has a generator that operates lights and a television," the dùgùtigi said. "The whole village watches it at night. Everyone knows Jackie Chan and his karate."

Now I understood the boys' fighting stances, yet I couldn't imagine the whole village crowded around a TV. No taking tea, no conversation, just silent faces staring at a blue screen under a black sky. There were other changes in Nampossela, as well. Two new foot-powered water pumps endlessly toiled at either end of the village, and a small store sold batteries, canned goods, candy, polyester shirts, and gasoline. Trash, mostly flimsy plastic bags and wrappers, gathered in corners and along walls. Ah, progress.

The clinic door was open. Henri Traoré was inside, speaking with a patient. I waited. I'd told him I wanted to see the clinic records Monique kept and anything else that might give me a better understanding of her time here since I'd left.

"Fatumata, please come in," Henri said in a rich, almost formal voice as the woman left.

Of all the villagers, Henri had changed the most. His cherubic features had matured into a degree of stateliness and he'd gained quite a few kilos. A new blue moped was parked outside the clinic, waiting to transport him the short distance to his home.

"Welcome back," Henri said as he sat down at Monique's desk. He crossed his legs, lifted one foot, and rested it on the other polyester-clad knee. His hefty legs strained the pants fabric, erasing the carefully ironed crease. He smiled at me kindly.

I took a seat just inside the doorway, always my favorite spot. A breeze passed in the door and out the window, offering the slightest relief from the heat. The clinic was in moderate disarray, but well stocked. There were two medicine cabinets now and they were stuffed with bottles and boxes. Containers were piled underneath Monique's old desk, and in the corner was a tumble of pills, cotton swabs, and syringes.

Henri reached back into a trunk, retrieving two ledgers. I settled the thick books, swathed in dark green fabric, on my lap. *Registre de Consultations Prenatales* and *Registre d'Accouchements*. Records of Monique's prenatal consultations and the births she attended.

"You know, Monique was even interviewed for the radio. The station in Koutiala talked to her about her work as a midwife. It aired on the radio in the weeks before she died."

Monique, the local celebrity, the beloved midwife. Yet she was not considered a midwife by international standards. Her nine months of medical training to become a matrone never qualified her as a midwife per se, or even gave her the title of "skilled attendant." To become a midwife or *sage-femme* (wise-woman) would have taken two to four years of medical schooling.

I opened the ledgers and flipped through their lined pages. They covered the past two years of her work. From what I could glean from the numbers and names swirled in blue ink, Monique was doing over forty prenatal consultations every week. In recent years, Monique had averaged ten to twelve births a month; she attended her last mother one week before her own death. She had written me recently about her workload:

> For us, it is the work that kills us here. I have too much work at the maternity ward. Truly, there is a huge increase again, Fatumata. You know how many villages come for my prenatal consultations? 6 villages plus Nampossela makes 7 villages. You can imagine each month how many people. I can have 140 per month and also each month I can birth more than 10. It is so tiring without stop. Everyone runs to find me. Even if I come to Koutiala they come to find me for their births, you see? Fatumata, I am tired, the work is too much.

I closed the ledgers and kept them in my lap, her writing and work a welcome weight.

"Oui," Henri said, sucking in his breath. "Fatumata, ever since she started working in Nampossela, her work was too much. You cannot do this work without inconveniences. She suffered, I think."

He stopped and stared out the door, folded his hands on the desk. Near his plump entwined fingers were grooves of familiar writing—*Gentamicin, Kinimax 5cc, 114, 32*. Monique had the habit of writing directly on the desktop: names of medicines to buy at the pharmacy in Koutiala, numbers to enter in her ledgers, and the spare-moment doodles of a mind wandering through other worlds, pushed into the wood.

"There were many difficulties in her marriage, as well," Henri said. His tone lightened as he spoke of her personal life. "The husband has a large garden, but did not allow Monique to have anything from it. Yet she took care of both their families, hers and her in-laws'. The responsibility that should have been her husband's became Monique's. Maxim wanted her to seek divorce, to leave here and do her work in another village. But, in the end, she could not do it. She would have had to leave the children and would never have been happy with that."

Henri unfolded his hands, rose from his seat and gazed through the doorway toward the fields.

"Well, it was an act of God," he said. "What we can say is that we hope the earth will be light on her, where she now rests. She could not stay here any longer. That is all."

John and I walked through the village on our last evening in Nampossela. The position of Orion's Belt on the edge of the sky told me it was not yet late. We were headed to the family compound. We'd lobbied hard for the children's education and tonight Louis would decide.

Just ahead, the belotte players sat around their ramshackle table. A man with his back toward us turned and looked over his shoulder—it was Adama, his sharp features the same. We exchanged awkward night greetings. The others mumbled from behind their cards. It was as if they had aged on this very spot, except there were no fawning females. As older men, they either no longer attracted them or were no longer interested. Though I can't forget the struggle we had over Monique's salary, I felt for Adama. Nampossela was for him, as for Monique, the end of the road.

At Louis', John and I sat beside Amadou. We waited in silence for the men to come out of the hut. I could only imagine how hard it would be for Louis to let go of his last grandchild still residing in Nampossela, for Basil to join his sisters in Koutiala. It was not just on a practical work level that Basil would be missed, but on an emotional level as well. If he experienced greener pastures, he might never return.

Gawssou, the dùgùtigi, and Louis finally emerged.

"We have come to agreement." The dùgùtigi laughed and smiled a little as he spoke, eyes still lowered. "Louis has given his okay."

I suppressed my urge to jump up and hug them. I realized that François had given us, and Monique, a gift—he had not stood in the way of his children's schooling. Outside the compound, the grand fête, held in our honor, was just beginning. John and I would dance, to the delight of the villagers, I was sure. If only Monique could have joined us.

Our good-byes the next day were much the same as when we first left Nampossela; the elders came out and gave us good wishes for the road, Gawssou never left John's side, and François showed up and asked us to remind Julie (the volunteer who came after me) that she promised him a guitar.

But we were surprised to see Mawa. She was as large and quietly jolly as ever, perhaps more so, and with no baby on her back. The dùgùtigi carried a small stand with two flags, one Malian and the other the United States, a long ago gift from my parents. He must have kept them in a special place, for their colors were not faded.

"I want you to see my sons."

Mawa and the dùgùtigi stepped aside to reveal Lassiné and Fousseni. They were clad in identical Western-style jogging suits, proving that dressing twins in matching clothes was a universal, if unfortunate, inclination. They greeted us with small handshakes and polite grins. The dùgùtigi sat down on a nearby bench, flanked by his sons, held the flags in front of him and straightened his back. He wanted a photo. Mawa shook her head, too shy, and retreated behind us. John captured them on film, identical young faces of Nampossela's next generation on either side of an ancient one.

Back in Koutiala, Amadou, our intermediary, invited us to his family's compound. He had something to say to us in private. His siblings and cousins were watching a blaring TV balanced upon a wobbly table. The three of us sat close to them, but facing away from the loud, tinny entertainment.

"François came to see me last night in the village," Amadou said, his voice direct and polite. "He talked about the problems between the two families. And he wanted for me to tell you. He said, 'Voilà, Amadou, these people are the friends of Monique. I am the husband of Monique. If these people should be close to anyone in the village it is to me. Monique was a woman who had a lot of success. This success was a source of wickedness in the village. The villagers did everything so that Monique and I would not get along.'"

"What?" I stared in disbelief.

"François told me that the village men did not want Monique there. Monique was from Koutiala; she was like a foreigner. They did everything so the marriage would rot. They went to a féticheur who made it so that François and Monique would not get along. One day François found, hidden in a papaya tree in his garden, rotten meat. Just like that, what was inside the fruit from his papayas and his banana trees? All rot."

How much of this was true, I wondered? Féticheurs, good and bad, still practiced their faith, but I didn't believe them to be the source of

Monique's marital problems. I also knew that she had the greatest defense against their curses, even by Malian standards; she didn't believe them.

Amadou continued.

"Monique's family here in Koutiala knew that Monique suffered in her life. François claims that the parents of Monique said that he didn't love her and that, very sincerely, was false. He said if he did not love his wife, she would never be pregnant. He said, 'They do not understand that it is my wife that is dead, the mother of my children. I suffer as well.'"

I bit my tongue at the thought. He felt Monique's pregnancy was the result of their love?

"We must remember that François is the person responsible for the kids," Amadou said. "Louis is getting very old, soon he will be able to do nothing, eh? François told me something. He said that everyone in the village says that he, François, doesn't work. He said that they are wrong because what he has in his garden, many people do not have. He did it with his own bare hands. He did it for his children."

"He's lying," I growled, and told him of my conversation with Henri Traoré and the fact that François would not share his produce with Monique.

Amadou slowed his speech as he tried to find the right words to respond.

"Maybe he wishes he himself could attain what Monique had. François said that you have done nothing bad. On the contrary, what you wanted was only the best. But since Monique came back from the U.S.A., he has not had any peace. Monique had a strong personality, she had a lot of class, she was held in much esteem . . . truthfully, her husband *should* be envious."

"Do you think that we did a bad thing in bringing Monique to the States?" John asked.

Hot feelings of guilt made my clothes itch and feel too tight. I leaned back in my chair and stared skyward. I didn't want to know. I didn't want to know that I made her life any harder than it had already been.

"*Non*. It was not a bad thing for Monique. And it was not a bad thing for all the people who loved Monique. But for François . . . his wife was educated, had so many friends and relations; all of this and then she gets to go all the way to the United States of America. Her husband just closed up."

What if she had married Pascal? I wondered.

"So, Fatumata and Bakary, the reason I wanted to talk to you is to tell you that in terms of the children, we want François to arrive at loving them. Monique is at peace. You who are here try to make peace. For the sake of the children. François said he understood and that, if it pleases God, he will not deceive us."

It was a crowded Sunday after mass at the Catholic church in Koutiala. It was here where Monique's children would be going to school, the same one that Monique had attended when she was a girl. Here, Yvonne had started the process that led to Monique marrying her younger brother, moving to Nampossela, and becoming a midwife.

The walls of this church had witnessed the multitudes who'd come to Monique's funeral. Just to the south, and a stone's throw away, was the hospital where Monique had birthed four children, and where she'd died. To the east was the children's graveyard where two of her children were buried, her first son and her last, and beyond that was Monique's gravesite.

John and I were here, in the church courtyard, with Monique's younger sister Angele. At twenty-four, Angele was almost the exact age Monique was when I met her. Flippy-floppy in a coordinated way, she was always jogging or at least walking fast. When Angele grabbed our hands, she shook them as she would shake out wet laundry. I looked down at her flapping duck feet: Monique's feet, Dembele feet.

"Where are Christini and Gené?" I asked.

"They are here somewhere," Angele replied in her husky voice.

I looked around at the swarms of mothers, fathers, and running children. The mother in me was a little alarmed. Angele picked up on my reaction.

"Fatumata, they are fine."

I searched the crowd.

"Christini, come here," Angele called out into a group of children, grabbing at the air with her fingers.

I heard giggling. Christini turned, trying to escape as little hands conspired to push her in my direction. She slipped though their grasp, laughing and screaming, and ran off. The bystanders moved aside so I could keep an eye on her. Seeing that no one was in pursuit, she stopped, turned, and watched from a distance. The fingers of her left hand were in her mouth.

"Christini!" I called.

"Christini, come here!" Angele yelled with mock anger. "She is crazy, that one."

The other kids seemed to take this as a challenge, that they too could be crazy, and they began talking, chasing each other, and running amuck. Christini was lost in the tumult.

John and I were given chairs and told to sit so that we could eat, in celebration of the inauguration of a new priest. One of Monique's brothers, Joseph, the former acolyte who had much admired our motorcycle, sat down beside us. Serious and thoughtful at twenty-years-old, he was well on his way to becoming a priest himself, just as Monique had predicted.

Suddenly, something pulled my hair. I brushed my head, afraid of what oversize creature might have fallen or flown into me, and turned around. Christini dashed away into the throngs, stifling giggles. I bet this was what Monique was like as a child, mischievous and daring.

"There is your Christini," Angele said with a laugh, "and here is Gené."

Gené was no longer impish and rotund. She was quiet and tall, with striking features, her mother's looks and her father's height. It was hard to believe she used to joke so heartily and openly about all things flatulent. Her greetings were heavy. I looked at Gené's feet as she sat beside us. She wore plastic high heels, much too big for her. She noticed my gaze.

"A woman traded me for my sandals," she said in a small voice, "so she could walk home. These are hers."

Gené said she'd accompany us back to the compound when we were ready. She got up, making choppy, awkward steps in the huge shoes, and almost tripped. Then she slung each shoe into her left hand and walked away barefoot.

I was not interested in staying to eat and chat. All day I'd thought about visiting Monique's grave, and I was ready to go. John, Angele, and Joseph consented. We began our walk, away from Christini and Gené, away from the crowds, and onto the worn trail into the brush. We ascended the same small rise that Monique pointed out to me long ago, the hill on which generations of her family were buried.

We had spoken about François and his promises. Digested his words and explanations. Everyone was tepidly hopeful that he would become the father that the children needed.

"All is okay now," Angele said. "What has happened was meant to be. Fatumata and Bakary, you must know, there were many signs before Monique died, that the end was near. First, our mother Jeanne fell ill: a very bad sign. Then, Monique would look at me and at Jeanne as if she had never seen us before. As if she saw through us."

Angele imitated her sister, making a quizzical, almost pained expression, eyes open wide like a puppy that had unknowingly bitten its own tail.

"And after she died, the rains began. That day was just like today has been, sunny and hot. But the moment that Monique died, the sky became black. *Black.* It growled as if it would kill another person. We brought her body to the house. We washed her and wrapped her in white cloth. The sky kept getting darker. It rained and rained and rained. Thundered." Angele's voice rose in intensity and volume and her hands beat at the sky. "The rains started that day and didn't stop. The twentieth of September was the last rain we had before this day, the fifteenth of October. The people had already harvested. The millet was drying outside. This is very, very rare."

John and I stared at each other, agape. We had never heard of a rain coming so late.

"The family compound was full of people," Angele said. "Even at eleven at night! The room, the yard, even outside. The people came from all over. The next day, the church held hundreds at the funeral. Many, many mopeds came to the church that day. And even six cars."

Joseph continued the story, raising his hands, palms up, "We prayed, and after the prayer we brought her body to the cemetery. After the burial, we all came back to the family compound. We sang hymns of praise. The midwives who work in Koutiala and other towns came, as well as their bosses. This is how it was. This is how the people were. Her tomb was still fresh and all the people began to talk about who Monique was; they said that Monique listened to everyone, no matter who they were. That is what happened. The fact that we saw these things happen is enough. Certainly the coming of the rain is enough."

I felt oddly awake, invigorated by the words of Monique's siblings. Despite the heat, the earth felt cool as we strolled in and out of the shade. The four of us moved to the same rhythm as our feet slid across the sand . . . swish, plock, swish, plock.

"You must know that I will continue my sister's work," Angele said. "I will enroll in nursing school next year to become a midwife, *ni Allah sonna*—God willing."

She looked over at me, arms pumping, head up, giving no sign that she was a woman in mourning. And in her soft face full of determination, I saw Monique.

We were surrounded by earthen lumps worn smooth and hard from the seasons. Nestled under trees and between bushes, in pairs and by themselves. A few were topped with small crosses or had simple markers: rocks and calabashes. I saw two long concrete rectangles ahead of us, and Angele guided us to one of them. There was no inscription, just a welded metal cross at one end.

"This is Monique's. As you can see, her grave is quite nice."

It was actually pretty ugly, but its simplicity was appropriate. We just stared and I wiped my eyes. John did the same, and Joseph reminded us not to be sad. John reached into his pocket and pulled out the silver ring he'd been carrying since the States to give to Monique. He took a stick, dug deep beside the concrete, and buried it. Standing, he touched the new silver ring on his left hand then took out another from his pocket. The ring on his finger was from me, a gift for his thirty-fifth birthday two days earlier, and the one in his pocket was another of Monique's.

"Monique, I'm giving you this ring for the one you lost. It's to replace Pascal's ring. Thank you for being a good friend and an inspiration. And thank you for *your* ring—I know it was yours because it's so gaudy. May your resting place be cool."

A Malian farewell. John did not have Monique's hand to hold while he talked to her, but the ring seemed an appropriate substitute. He stood up and I took his place.

I patted where John just dug and ran the dirt between my fingertips. Grains of earth settled around the edges of Monique's ring on my right finger. Some fell into my palm, red and dull, with a few tiny glittering specks. Just dirt, but part of the land that would carry forth Angele's calling, grow François' garden and hopefully his heart, and feed Monique's children. My fingers followed the edge of the large flat marker that seemed to rise up from the ground itself. It was the size and shape of the old birthing table in Nampossela and so solid, so anchored, that I could imagine it with roots, as if it had sprouted and grown instead of having been framed and poured by human hands. Its straight angles blended with the roll of the hills and the eroded grave mounds. Only a few months old and already part of the landscape. It glowed white beneath the trees, under the watch of quiet sun.

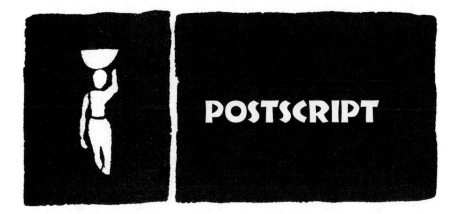

POSTSCRIPT

IT IS JANUARY 2006. I sit in the dry furnace-generated warmth of my New England home amid a landscape of short days and utter cold and marvel that my outside world ever held heat and green and noisy life. I look out at the white stillness and blue shadows and imagine motion—a group of Minianka women gathered around their mortars, pounding millet for breakfast as they talk and sway under Nampossela's night sky. A world away. And yet, if I wrap myself in a mudcloth blanket, submerge myself in the music of Habib Koité, or open a letter written in Bambara-laden French, Mali comes rushing in, and I experience a brief state of equilibrium when both worlds are home at once.

I keep in touch with Nampossela, mostly through Henri Traoré. He's a frequent writer and remains the village health worker in what continues to be a thriving clinic. The maternity ward is still standing—a small miracle after all these years—and more importantly, continues to provide care and shelter for birthing women. A new midwife was hired a few years back (Monique's apprentice Koniba never finished her training). She is not from the village, but nonetheless is Minianka. The dùgùtigi, Mawa, and Gawssou are well, just older and slower. The Peace Corps sporadically places a volunteer in Nampossela. Henri couldn't say if or when the next one might arrive.

Louis died in 2001, leaving François as head of the family. Henri wrote that François took another wife, though he didn't give her name or say if they have children. For years after our last visit, John and I followed Amadou's advice. We diligently wrote François. We asked about the family, his garden, and the village, until his lack of response withered our commitment to put pen to paper.

François has kept his promise of not standing in the way of his children's education. Through the great support of Monique's parents and siblings, and the financial support of friends and family in the States, Christini, Basil, and Gené all attend school. We stay in touch through e-mail, which two of Monique's brothers have, and an occasional cell phone call. Basil and Gené now live with one of Monique's brothers and his family in Bamako. Louis was right—Basil will never return to Nampossela. Christini lives with Angele, who finished her degree in midwifery and is now completing her internship. Angele continues her sister's work.

Monique's brother Joseph attends seminary and will be ordained as a priest in 2007. The family plans a huge celebration. John and I hope to return to Mali at this time, and to bring Aidan and Liam along. Jeanne and Apollinaire have long said that the absence of their "white grandchildren" is unacceptable.

Maxim, Monique's eldest cousin, recently opened a rural clinic near Nampossela in Monique's honor, affectionately named *Cabinet de soins Monique*. The clinic, when fully operational, will offer medical consultations, perform minor surgeries, and have gynecological and obstetrical care. When Angele finishes her training, she plans to work here. A portion of the proceeds of this book will go to support Monique's children's health and education and to provide capital (a new building, materials, equipment) and program development at this clinic.

Of course, I still miss Monique, and I wonder what the rest of her life would have held for her. I think she would have been thrilled at Mali's successful democracy and at the growing number of women's groups that address girls' education, maternal and child health, and female genital cutting. She would have been a part of this change; I hope her children will be. And I hope that as women gain more rights and enjoy more choices in Mali these changes will only add color and strength to Malian community life, providing ample room for women to make their homes within it.

BIBLIOGRAPHY AND RECOMMENDED READING

AbouZahr, C., T. Wardlaw, C. Stanton, and K. Hill. "Maternal Mortality." *World Health Statistics Quarterly* 49, no. 2 (1996): 77–87.

Allen, Denise. *Managing Motherhood, Managing Risk: Fertility and Danger in West Central Tanzania.* Ann Arbor: University of Michigan Press, 2004.

Ba, Mariama. *So Long a Letter.* Oxford: Heinemann, 1980.

Barnes, Virginia Lee, and Janice Boddy. *Aman: The Story of a Somali Girl.* New York: Random House, 1994.

Bates, Daniel G., and Elliot M. Fratkin. *Cultural Anthropology.* Boston: Allyn & Bacon, 1999.

Burns, A. August, Ronnie Lovich, Jane Maxwell, and Katharine Shapiro. *Where Women Have No Doctor: A Health Guide for Women.* Berkeley: The Hesperian Foundation, 2000.

Caldwell, John C. *Theory of Fertility Decline.* London: Academic Press, 1982.

Castle, Sarah E. "Intra-Household Differentials in Women's Status: Household Function and Focus as Determinants of Children's Illness Management and Care in Rural Mali." *Health Transition Review* 3, no. 2 (1993): 137–157.

Center for Reproductive Rights and Association des Jurists Maliennes. *Claiming Our Rights: Surviving Pregnancy and Childbirth in Mali.* New York: Center for Reproductive Rights and Association des Jurists Maliennes, 2003.

Cleland, John G., and Jerome K. Van Ginneken. "Maternal Education and Child Survival in Developing Countries: The Search for Pathways of Influence." *Soc. Sci. Med.* 27, no. 12 (1988): 1357–1368.

Clifford, James, and George E. Marcus, eds. *Writing Culture: The Poetics and Politics of Ethnography.* Berkeley: University of California Press, 1986.

De Brouwere V., R. Tonglet, and W. Van Lerberghe. "Strategies for Reducing Maternal Mortality in Developing Countries: What Can We Learn from the History of the Industrialized West?" *Tropical Medicine and International Health* 3, no. 10 (1998): 771–782.

Davidson, Basil. *A History of West Africa: 1000–1800.* Essex: Longman. 1985.
———. *West Africa Since 1800: The Revolutionary Years.* Essex: Longman, 1986.
Davis-Floyd, Robbie, and Carolyn Sargent. *Childbirth and Authoritative Knowledge.* Berkeley: University of California Press, 1997
Dettwyler, Katherine A. *Dancing Skeletons: Life and Death in West Africa.* Long Grove, IL: Waveland Press, 1994.
Diallo, Yaya, and Mitchell Hall. *The Healing Drum: African Wisdom Teachings.* Rochester, VT: Destiny Books, 1989.
Earl, Scott, ed. *Life Before the Drought.* Boston: Allen & Unwin, 1984.
Direction Nationale de la Statistique et de l'Informatique. *Enquête Démographique et de Santé, Mali, 1995–1996.* Bamako, Mali: Direction Nationale de la Statistique et de l'Informatique, 1996.
Etard, J. F., B. Kodio, and S. Traore. "Assessment of Maternal Mortality and Late Maternal Mortality among a Cohort of Pregnant Women in Bamako, Mali." *British Journal of Obstetrics & Gynaecology* 106, no. 1 (1999): 60–65.
Federici, Nora, Karen Oppenheim Mason, and Solvi Sogner, eds. *Women's Position and Demographic Change.* Oxford: Clarendon, 1993.
Freire, Paulo. *Pedagogy of the Oppressed.* New York: Continuum, 1970.
Gilligan, Carol. *In a Different Voice.* Cambridge, MA: Harvard University Press, 1982.
Gottlieb, Alma, and Philip Graham. *Parallel Worlds: An Anthropologist and a Writer Encounter Africa.* Chicago: University of Chicago Press, 1993.
Gruenbaum, Ellen. *The Female Circumcision Controversy: An Anthropological Perspective.* Philadelphia: University of Pennsylvania Press, 2001.
Hill, Allan G., and D. F. Roberts, eds. "Health Interventions and Mortality Change in Developing Countries." *Journal of Biosocial Science,* Suppl. no. 10, Cambridge: Parkes Foundation (1989): 1–136.
Hoestermann C. F., G. Ogbaselassie, J. Wacker, and G. Bastert. "Maternal Mortality in the Main Referral Hospital in The Gambia, West Africa." *Tropical Medicine and International Health* 1, no. 5 (1996): 710–717.
Howson, Christopher P., Polly F. Harrison, Dana Hotra, and Maureen Law, eds. *In Her Lifetime: Female Morbidity and Mortality in Sub-Saharan Africa.* Washington, DC: National Academy Press, 1996.
Hunt, Nancy Rose. *A Colonial Lexicon of Birth Ritual, Medicalization, and Mobility in the Congo.* Durham, NC: Duke University, 1999.
Imperata, Pascal James. *Historical Dictionary of Mali.* Metuchen, NJ: Scarecrow Press, 1977.
Jordan, Brigitte. *Birth in Four Cultures: A Crosscultural Investigation of Childbirth in Yucatan, Holland, Sweden, and the United States.* Long Grove, IL: Waveland Press, 1993
Kassindja, Fauziya, and Layli Miller Bashir. *Do They Hear You When You Cry?* New York: Delacorte Press, 1998.
Klein, Susan. *A Book for Midwives: A Manual for Traditional Birth Attendants and Community Midwives.* Berkeley: Hesperian Foundation, 1995.

Koblinksy, M. A. et al. "Organizing Delivery Care: What Works for Safe Motherhood?" *Bulletin of the World Health Organization* 77, no. 5 (1999): 399–406.

Kynch, Jocelyn, and Amartya Sen. "Indian Women: Well-Being and Survival." *Cambridge Journal of Economics,* no. 7 (1983): 363–380.

Lee, K. S., S. C. Park, B. Khoshnood, H. L. Hsieh, and R. Mittendorf. "Human Development Index as a Predictor of Infant and Maternal Mortality Rates." *Journal of Pediatrics* 131, no. 3 (1997): 430–433.

Leonardo, Micaela di, ed. *Gender at the Crossroads of Knowledge: Feminist Anthropology in the Postmodern Era.* Berkeley: University of California Press, 1991.

Leslie, J., and G. R. Gupta. *Utilization of Formal Services for Maternal Nutrition and Health Care in the Third World.* Washington, DC: International Center for Research on Women, 1989.

Liljestrand, J., and W. G. Povey, eds. *Maternal Health Care in an International Perspective.* Uppsala, Sweden: Dept. Of Obstetrics and Gynaecology, Uppsala University, and World Health Organization, 1992.

Mabila, Mara. *Breast Feeding and Sexuality: Behaviour, Beliefs, and Taboos among the Gogo Mothers in Tanzania.* New York: Berghahn Books, 2005.

Mason, Karen Oppenheim. "The Impact of Women's Social Position on Fertility in Developing Countries." *Sociological Forum* 2, no. 4 (1987): 718–745.

————. *The Status of Women: A Review of Its Relationships to Fertility and Mortality.* Population Studies Center, University of Michigan. Paper for the Population Sciences Division of the Rockefeller Foundation, 1984.

Mathabane, Mark. *African Women: Three Generations.* New York: HarperCollins, 1994.

Merchant, K., and R. Martorell. "Frequent Reproductive Cycling: Does It Lead to Nutritional Depletion of Mothers?" *Progress in Food and Nutrition Science,* no. 12 (1988): 339–369.

Mitford, Jessica. *The American Way of Birth.* New York: Dutton, 1992.

PATH (Program for Appropriate Technology in Health). "Safe Motherhood: Successes and Challenges." *Outlook* 16, Special Issue (July 1998): 1–2.

Paulme, Denise, ed. *Women of Tropical Africa,* Berkeley: University of California Press, 1963

Pinstrup-Andersen, Per, David Pelletier, and Harold Alderman, eds. *Child Growth and Nutrition in Developing Countries: Priorities for Action.* Ithaca: Cornell University Press,1995.

Riesman, Paul. *Freedom in Fulani Social Life: An Introspective Ethnography.* Chicago: University of Chicago Press, 1974.

Rogers, Susan Carol. "Woman's Place: A Critical Review of Anthropological Theory." *Comparative Studies in Society and History* 20 (1978): 123–162.

Romney, Patricia, Beverly Tatum, and JoAnne Jones. "Feminist Strategies for Teaching about Oppression: The Importance of Process." *Women's Studies Quarterly* 20, nos. 1 & 2 (1992): 95–110.

Sagara, A. A. *Légendes du Mali,* Bamako, Mali: Éditions Jamana, 1990.

Sargent, Carolyn. *The Cultural Context of Therapeutic Choice: Obstetrical Care Decisions among the Bariba of Benin.* Dordrecht: D. Reidel, 1982.

———. *Maternity, Medicine, and Power: Reproductive Decisions in Urban Benin.* Berkeley: University of California Press, 1989.

Stamm, Liesa, and Carol D. Ryff. *Social Power and Influence of Women.* Boulder, CO: Westview, 1984.

Stewart, M. Kathryn, Cynthia K. Stanton, and Omar Ahmed. "Maternal Health Care." *Demographic and Health Surveys Comparative Studies,* no. 25. Calverton, MD: Macro International, 1997.

Tinker, Irene, ed. *Persistent Inequalities: Women and World Development.* New York: Oxford University Press, 1990.

Toulmin, Camilla. *Cattle, Women, and Wells: Managing Household Survival in the Sahel.* Oxford: Clarendon Press, 1992.

Van Esterik, Penny. *Beyond the Breast-Bottle Controversy.* New Brunswick, NJ: Rutgers University Press, 1989.

Velton, Ross. *Mali: The Bradt Travel Guide.* Bucks, UK: Bradt, 2000.

World Bank. *World Development Report 1993: Investing in Health.* Washington, DC: World Bank, 1993.

Young, Kate, Carol Wolkowitz, and Roslyn McCullagh, eds. *Of Marriage and the Market: Women's Subordination in International Perspective.* London: CSE Books, 1981.

Web Sites

Safe Motherhood—www.safemotherhood.org, www.matercare.org

Reproductive Health Outlook—www.rho.org

United Nations Population Fund—www.unfpa.org

Center for Reproductive Rights and Research—www.crlp.org

Demographic and Health Surveys, Mali DHS Surveys—www.measuredhs.com

The Centre for Development and Population Activities (CEDPA)—www.cedpa.org

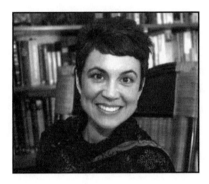

Kris Holloway served as a Peace Corps volunteer in Mali, West Africa, 1989–1991, where she met her husband John Bidwell. She holds an MPH from the University of Michigan. She currently works with the Center for International Studies, a study abroad organization (www.cisabroad.com) and lives in Northampton, MA, with John, their two sons, and one giant poodle.

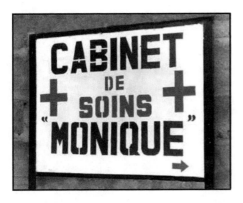

In 2004, Maxim Dembele, a village health worker and Monique's favorite cousin, founded the rural health clinic, Cabinet de Soins Monique (or Clinique Monique), in Monique's honor. The clinic is located in Kouri, a small town in Mali with a population of roughly 5,000 on the Burkino Faso border—just east of Koutiala, where Monique was born, and Nampossela, where Monique worked. The purpose of the clinic is to conduct prenatal consultations, perform minor surgeries, and provide gynecological and obstetrical care.

Proceeds from the sales of *Monique and the Mango Rains* will help expand the capabilities of this clinic, as well as provide school-tuition assistance and health care for Monique's children.

Examples of what donations can do:
- $1,000 pays for one solar generator and back-up battery
- $300 pays for one year of midwifery training
- $100 sends a child to school for one year
- $50 pays for a set of obstetrical instruments

We are partnered with WomensTrust, Inc., a 501c3 nonprofit organization dedicated to empowering women in West Africa at the grassroots level. Donations to Clinique Monique are tax deductible and urgently needed to make Maxim's dream of expanding this clinic a reality. Donations may be made securely online through PayPal at www.moniquemangorains.com on the "How to Help" page or by mailing a check payable to "Clinique Monique" to WomensTrust, Inc., P.O. Box 15, Wilmot, NH 03287

For more information about this project, please e-mail us at cliniquemonique@moniquemangorains.com

Our utmost thanks.

Kris Holloway and John Bidwell